Keeping the Blues Away

THE TEN-STEP GUIDE TO REDUCING THE RELAPSE OF DEPRESSION

CATE HOWELL CSM

Illustrations by

DR SUSAN WORBOYS AND ALEX BARNARD

Radcliffe Publishing
Oxford • New York

Radcliffe Publishing Ltd
18 Marcham Road
Abingdon
Oxon OX14 1AA
United Kingdom

www.radcliffe-oxford.com

Electronic catalogue and worldwide online ordering facility.

British Library Cataloguing in Publication Data

A catalogue record for this book is available from the British Library.

ISBN-13: 978 184619 372 9

The paper used for the text pages of this book is FSC certified. FSC (The Forest Stewardship Council) is an international network to promote responsible management of the world's forests.

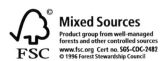

Mixed Sources
Product group from well-managed forests and other controlled sources
www.fsc.org Cert no. SGS-COC-2482
© 1996 Forest Stewardship Council

Typeset by Pindar NZ, Auckland, New Zealand
Printed and bound by TJI Digital, Padstow, Cornwall, UK

369 0028934

2010

Keeping the Blues Away

X

Contents

Preface

In 2004, a study of a primary care treatment program aiming to reduce the severity and relapse of depression was begun. The treatment program was called *Keeping the Blues Away* (KBA) and involved active therapy and monitoring over 12 months. A ten-step program was developed and its effectiveness studied in 100 individuals with depression. The aim was to reduce severity and relapse of depression over a 12-month period.

The KBA program was based on clinical experience and research which suggested that a novel multifaceted program including psychological and social aspects was needed. A 200-page treatment manual and relaxation tracks were developed and used by General Practitioners (GPs) who guided participants with depression through the program.

The study demonstrated that KBA was a promising program, and the results have been published in the *Medical Journal of Australia* (www.mja.com). KBA has the potential to help many individuals with depression to become well and remain well. The program was received positively by the GPs and their patients. GPs commented that they believed many people with both anxiety and depression could benefit from the program.

The treatment guide and relaxation tracks, available at www.radcliffe-oxford. com/keepingthebluesaway, are now being published. It is suggested that the individual works through KBA in regular consultation with a GP or mental health professional (MHP), such as a psychologist, mental health social worker, occupational therapist or counsellor. The clinician can adapt the program to suit the individual by focusing on particular aspects, or adding other materials. An introduction to this guide is provided for clinicians. However, the guide and tracks may also be used by the individual as a self-help tool to self-manage the depression. Further information on the program is available from www.keepingthebluesaway.com.

Cate Howell
September 2009

Acknowledgements

This guide would not have been possible without help from a number of people. For their support and assistance, I would like to thank:

Professor Justin Beilby
Dr Sheila Clark
Professor Ian Wilson
Teresa Burgess
Professor Chris Dowrick
Professor Jonathan Newbury
Dr Marion Bailes
Dr Samira Peera
Melissa Opolski

Professor John Marley
Dr Fiona Hawker
Dr Nigel Stocks
Dr Ruth Walker
Professor Deb Turnbull
Wendy Newbury
Dr Jim Barnard
Dr Michele Murphy
Joseph Hinora

Many thanks to the following organisations for their support of the study:

Royal Australian College of General Practitioners
The University of Adelaide
Primary Health Care Research, Evaluation and Development Program
Spencer Gulf Rural Health School
beyondblue, the national depression initiative

A number of participants and their partners read the guide and provided feedback. They shall remain anonymous, but their input was invaluable.

I would especially like to thank Dr Susan Worboys and Alex Barnard for the illustrations, and Ada Lester for her enthusiasm, help and creativity in producing the guide.

Introduction to this guide for clinicians

The desire to develop a depression treatment program which addresses the whole person (including biological, psychosocial and spiritual facets) stemmed from years of providing clinical care for individuals with depression. A Churchill Fellowship provided the opportunity to travel to the United Kingdom and Europe to investigate the primary care management of depression and anxiety. There was consensus amongst leaders in the field that the primary care management of depression including relapse prevention was an important area to investigate further. As a result, the *Keeping the Blues Away* (KBA) program, which aims to reduce the severity of depression and prevent relapse, was developed.

Segal, Williams, and Teasdale (2002) suggest that it might be possible to take the active ingredients of proven treatments and design novel preventive treatments that are skills based (Segal, Williams, and Teasdale, 2002). KBA is a novel, multifaceted program, which draws on a number of evidence-based therapies, such as Cognitive-behavioural Therapy (CBT), Interpersonal Therapy (IPT), Acceptance and Commitment Therapy (ACT), Problem-Solving Therapy, Well-being Therapy and Mindfulness-based Cognitive Therapy. It is also influenced by Narrative and Existential Therapies.

KBA incorporates assessment, treatment planning, and regular follow-up of patients. It provides information and exercises to teach coping skills (e.g. stress management and problem solving), in addition to cognitive-behavioural and interpersonal skills, and relapse prevention strategies. KBA recognises the importance of involving family or carers wherever possible, using medication if clinically indicated and managing coexisting medical problems.

The efficacy of KBA in the general practice setting has been studied in a pilot randomised controlled trial. KBA was found to be a promising program for older patients in particular, and for those with more severe or persistent symptoms. KBA was positively received by GPs and patients. A paper on the rationale for the program, the results of the randomized controlled trial (RCT) and a further paper on management of recurrent depression and the role of KBA have been published

(Howell, 2004; Howell, Marshall, Opolski *et al.*, 2008; Howell, Turnbull, Beilby, *et al.*, 2008). The program is now being used in multidisciplinary mental health teams, and a further study is planned with mental health professionals (MHPs) delivering the program. A newly developed computer-assisted version of KBA has also been developed.

The KBA program is presented as a treatment manual that serves as a guide for the general practitioner (GP) or MHP, and also as a workbook for the individual with depression. The GP or MHP works collaboratively with the patient through the 10 steps of the KBA program. It is recommended that the program be commenced once the individual is able to concentrate and participate in a structured program. Regular appointments over a three-month period will be needed to cover the material in KBA, and the patient is then followed up regularly for 12 months or more.

To gain the best outcomes from KBA, do not rush through the program. Take small steps – each step of the program may take a number of sessions to cover. Provide some background to the relevance of each step, and help the patient begin some of the exercises during the sessions. If you are not familiar with the content of the step or the therapy it is based on, for example, CBT or IPT, it is helpful and important to access further information from text books, articles or courses to increase your knowledge and skill in the area.

The KBA program is set out in this manual in an easy-to-follow format, comprising 10 steps, each one covering key areas in depression management and relapse prevention. The clinician can guide the person through each step of the program. One step of the program builds on the next, for example, stress is introduced in Step 1, more detail is provided in Step 3, and strategies for managing stress are covered in the subsequent steps. Summary tables ('points to remember') are used to reinforce key information.

The 10 steps in the manual are as follows:
1. getting started: information about depression and anxiety, and relapse prevention
2. medical and psychosocial assessment, goal setting, monitoring progress
3. healthy lifestyle issues (nutrition, exercise, sleep, managing stress)
4. useful coping skills (mood diary, problem solving, relaxation techniques)
5. helpful thinking or cognitive strategies (thought monitoring, analysis and challenging)
6. dealing with psychological issues (self-esteem, loss and grief, anger and guilt, hopelessness and suicidal thoughts)
7. the benefits of activity (activity scheduling, laughter and humour)
8. fostering social support and skills, dealing with relationship issues and unemployment
9. developing a plan to manage early symptoms of relapse
10. reassessment, review and helpful resources.

The three relaxation tracks available at www.radcliffe-oxford.com/keepingthe bluesaway cover:

➤ general relaxation, including progressive muscle relaxation, breathing techniques and visualisation
➤ a colour meditation, which is ego-strengthening
➤ a mindfulness-based meditation.

The tracks are highlighted in Steps 4 and 5 in the program, as they fit with material covered in these steps. Patients are encouraged to listen to each of the tracks at different stages of the program, and to use them regularly.

Step 1 in KBA provides key information for patients and family members. Psycho-education is a vital part of treatment (Ellis and Royal Australian and New Zealand College of Psychiatrists Clinical Practice Team for Depression, 2004). Available treatments (medication and psychosocial) are explained, for example, use of medication and the range of psychological therapies. Anxiety is also addressed as it often coexists with depression (World Health Organization Centre for Mental Health and Substance Abuse, 2000).

Step 2 in the KBA manual provides a brief summary of assessment (medical and psychological) and also takes the individual through goal setting. It is best if the patient focuses on short-term goals early on, and these can be reviewed regularly. As improvement occurs, the individual will be able to set more medium-term or long-term goals. It is valuable to work on goals that are meaningful to the patient and fit with the patient's values (Harris, 2007).

Step 3 addresses healthy lifestyle issues, such as nutrition and exercise, and stress management. The information provided is based on commonsense and evidence, and can be tailored to the individual patient.

The treatment program teaches a number of useful coping skills including keeping a mood diary, problem solving and relaxation techniques. In Step 4 the patient is guided through each of these skills, and it will take a number of sessions – with work set between the sessions – to cover all the skills and apply them, such as putting problem solving into practice and using the relaxation tracks.

There is evidence for the effectiveness of CBT in treating depression and preventing relapse (Fava, Rafanelli, Grandi, et al., 1998; Jarrett, Kraft, Doyle, et al., 2001; Paykel, Scott, Teasdale, et al., 1999). Step 5 guides the individual through the principles of CBT in a novel way. 'Five steps to tackle unhelpful thinking that can occur in depression' have been outlined in this step, namely:

1. keeping a thought diary
2. understanding thinking errors
3. identifying thinking errors
4. challenging unhelpful thinking
5. developing more helpful thoughts.

Tables are provided for keeping a record for each of these stages. As with Step 4, this step will take a number of clinical sessions to work through. The person will begin keeping a thought diary at the start, and will look at thinking errors and challenging unhelpful thinking in subsequent sessions. The individual can be given tasks to do in between sessions.

Towards the end of Step 5, several important issues related to CBT for depression and the origin of thinking errors are covered. It is explained that individuals may develop assumptions and beliefs about the world, others and themselves. Beliefs operate at an unconscious level, and come into play when responding to situations (Blackburn and Davidson, 1995). During depression, an individual's beliefs tend to be more negative and unhelpful, and may include needing to obtain the approval of everyone around them, or needing to be 'perfect' at tasks (Blackburn and Davidson, 1995; Kidman, 2006). Strategies are then provided to assist the individual to develop more helpful beliefs (Greenberger and Padesky, 1995).

A section on mindfulness completes this step, as it is helpful in addressing negative thinking styles. Through paying purposeful attention to the present moment, mindfulness provides a way of raising awareness of one's thinking (Segal, Williams, and Teasdale, 2002; Teasdale, Segal, Williams, *et al.*, 2000). Increased awareness of negative thoughts allows a person to realise when they are about to undergo a downward mood swing. It has been suggested that being aware of this weakens the depressed thought, making it possible for the individual to halt the vicious cycle between negative thoughts and negative feelings (Segal, Williams, and Teasdale, 2002). A brief mindfulness-based meditation is provided at www.radcliffe-oxford.com/keepingthebluesaway.

An outline of the elements of Acceptance and Commitment Therapy (ACT) is included towards the end of Step 5.

Step 6 addresses a number of key psychological issues that may be experienced in depression. These are:
1. low self-esteem
2. loss and grief
3. the 'negative' emotions (anger and jealousy, guilt and shame)
4. difficulty letting go of negative emotions
5. loneliness and depression.
6. hopelessness, suicidal thoughts and depression
7. difficulty finding hope and meaning.

It is important to tailor this step for the individual, by identifying and focusing on the most relevant parts of the step. This step can be challenging and the patient may need extra support and time to work through the information and emotions provoked.

Activity is central to life. I qualified and practised as an Occupational Therapist (OT) before I trained as a doctor, and later as a GP. As an OT, I saw meaningful activity change people's lives for the better. Loss of motivation and lethargy are common in depression, which means that the individual is less likely to do the activities that usually provide them with pleasure. A vicious circle can result – the less active the individual becomes, the more depressed they feel and the less they do (Hickie, 2000; Kidman, 2006). Step 7 therefore looks at the benefits of activity and incorporates active scheduling of pleasurable activities. It also looks at the philosophy of keeping life simple, and at the benefits of laughter and humour.

Step 8 of KBA considers ways to foster social support and skills, as these are central to positive life experiences. This step is very much based on IPT, which emphasises the role of psychosocial difficulties in depression – interpersonal events can lead to depressive symptoms and the depression can impair a person's ability to function interpersonally (Davies, 2000; Sadock and Sadock, 2007). Step 8 therefore covers the importance of social connectedness and assertiveness skills. It also addresses relationship issues (including conflict), dealing with unemployment and identifying social supports.

It is recognised that it is important to develop a written depression-relapse prevention plan with the patient (Hickie, 2000). This involves helping the patient identify and record early warning symptoms (which might suggest a recurrence), and specific risk factors. It is important that the plan addresses the maintenance of physical health and strategies to reduce stress and anxiety. Step 9 takes the patient through the steps involved in developing an emergency plan for relapse, including targeting early warning symptoms and possible high-risk situations (Williams, 2000; World Health Organization Collaborating Centre for Mental Health and Substance Abuse, 2000).

At Step 10 of the program, the patient's progress will be reassessed. Steps 1 to 9 are reviewed, as repetition and reinforcement are important aspects of any psychosocial treatment program for depression. The GP or MHP can draw the patient's attention to the list of useful resources provided in the manual.

SUMMARY

I use KBA in my practice very regularly, and find it provides a helpful and user-friendly approach. It is worth familiarising yourself with the program in detail to enable you to work easily through the 10 steps. KBA is holistic and well accepted by patients. The KBA resources are easy to follow and understand, and yet cover the areas relevant to depression assessment and management. I hope that you and the individuals you are working with find KBA helpful as well.

Further information on the background to the program and associated research can be found in:

➤ Howell C. Preventing depression relapse: a primary care approach. *Prim Care Ment Health*. 2004; **2**: 151–6.
➤ Howell C, Turnbull D, Beilby J, *et al*. Preventing relapse of depression in primary care: a pilot study of the 'Keeping the blues away' program. *Med J Aust*. 2008; **188**(12 Suppl.): S138–41.
➤ Howell C, Marshall C, Opolski M, *et al*. Management of recurrent depression. *Aust Fam Physician*. 2008; **37**(9): 704–8.

Introduction

Welcome to the *Keeping the Blues Away* (KBA) program, which is presented as a written guide and relaxation tracks (available at www.radcliffe-oxford.com/keepingthebluesaway) to help you recover from depression and to stay well. It is based on current literature and research about depression, has developed out of work and study in Australia and overseas, and has been influenced by many years of clinical experience.

The program has been designed to be **holistic** in its approach, recognising that all aspects of a person's life are important. Most people want to be able to **function day to day** and find a sense of **quality of life** again. So the program aims to be very practical and oriented towards everyday life.

The KBA program incorporates treatment strategies that have been shown to be helpful in managing depression. Selecting what seem to be the most appropriate treatment strategies from a range of treatment methods is called an **eclectic** approach. It is commonly used in the general practice or primary healthcare setting, and allows the general practitioner (GP) or mental health professional (MHP) to offer the best treatment for the individual patient's needs.

The program involves 10 steps.

Step 1:   Getting started – information about depression.
Step 2:   Assessment and goal setting.
Step 3:   Healthy lifestyle issues.
Step 4:   Useful coping skills.
Step 5:   Helpful thinking or cognitive strategies.
Step 6:   Dealing with psychological issues.
Step 7:   The benefits of activity.
Step 8:   Fostering social support and skills.
Step 9:   Developing a plan to manage early relapse symptoms.
Step 10: Reassess and review, plus helpful resources.

Take one step at a time. There is flexibility in the program. As you work through the program, you and your GP or MHP can focus on areas of most importance for you. One step builds on the next step; for example, Step 1 talks about anxiety, and in Steps 3 and 4 there are specific skills for dealing with stress and anxiety.

It is really important for you to find ways to cope with the symptoms of depression, associated anxiety and with life stress. This program focuses on developing your understanding of depression and associated anxiety, as well as teaching **strategies to cope** and useful skills. It is about providing a resource, and developing the **resources** already within you, to manage depression and help prevent relapse.

Thank you for making a **commitment** to the program. As with many things in life, the program will bring most benefit with effort and work. Make a commitment to yourself to attend appointments, read the notes and do the exercises as you go along. Some of the work will be done with the GP or MHP, and some will need to be done in between sessions. Once you have developed strategies and skills, **persist** with them.

Using this written guide your GP or MHP will help you through the program and provide encouragement and **support** as you do so. Keep a note of questions in between appointments with your GP. Let them know if you have any problems with, or concerns about, the program.

It is recommended that you have an exercise book to use as a **journal**, as you may want to write down questions or concerns, or do some of the suggested exercises in it. It can be used to record your ideas, or experiences of the depression, treatment and recovery. Taking time to pause and jot down what you are thinking and feeling can be very important.

Getting started – information about depression

Or the *'who, what, why, how, when and where'* of depression and relapse!

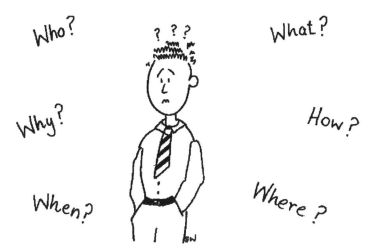

Your GP or MHP may have already talked with you and provided information about depression. Having information for yourself and your family to look at is really important in managing the depression. It can help you have a greater sense of **understanding and control**, which can be a very positive step towards recovery.

Some information may be repeated here, and other information may be new. Other ways to access more information in the community or via the internet will be outlined later (*see* Resources in Step 10).

WHO GETS DEPRESSED?

Depression is a common problem and can affect anyone – in fact, it will affect about 1 in 5 individuals at some time in their lives. It is experienced by males and females of all ages, but is more common in women. However, women with depression are more likely than men with depression to seek help from their doctor (Evans, Burrows and Norman, 2000; Hickie, 2002; Kessler, Berglund, Demler, *et al.*, 2003).

WHAT IS DEPRESSION?

➤ Everyone experiences feelings of sadness, loss or 'depressed' feelings at some time. These are part of life, and part of coming to terms with difficult events in life. But these common feelings are not the same as 'depression'.

➤ The term 'depression' is used to describe **a condition in which mood is persistently and severely depressed**. The low mood and other associated symptoms are debilitating, **affecting the ability to cope and function** (Evans, Burrows and Norman, 2000; Hickie, 2002).

➤ It can be very difficult to go to a GP or MHP and talk about feeling depressed. There are still a lot of myths about mental illness in our community and misconceptions about depression. These lead to stigma (Hickie, 2002). Depression **may be wrongly viewed as weakness**, and it may be thought that the person should, for example, just 'get over it'.

➤ Sometimes it is hard to pick that the problem is depression. It may seem that the main problem is tiredness or disturbed sleep. Often individuals go to the doctor with a physical problem, rather than recognising that there is an emotional concern. Another complication is that anxiety often accompanies depression, and may seem to dominate initially.

➤ The diagnosis of depression requires the following symptoms to be present.

For at least a two-week period, either consistently low or depressed mood, and/or loss of enjoyment or interest in most activities. At least four other key depressive symptoms will have been present:
- significant weight or appetite changes
- too little or too much sleep
- agitation or slowing down
- significant decrease in energy levels, or excessive tiredness
- feeling very guilty or worthless
- having trouble making decisions, thinking clearly, or concentrating
- thinking frequently about death or suicide.

(American Psychiatric Association, 2000.)

HOW DO I KNOW THAT I HAVE DEPRESSION?

Depression varies in severity, and symptoms may be mild, moderate or severe. Symptoms vary from person to person. The symptoms of depression **affect a person's thoughts, feelings and everyday functioning.** It can be helpful to think of the symptoms as being psychological and physical.

PSYCHOLOGICAL SYMPTOMS	PHYSICAL SYMPTOMS
Low mood, feelings of sadness	Sleep problems – finding it hard to get off to sleep, sleeping too much or too little
Loss of pleasure, interest	
Loss of motivation	Tiredness, low energy
Irritability	Physical aches and pains
Crying easily	Agitation or restlessness
Emotional numbness	Slowing down
Withdrawal from others	Appetite/weight changes
Anxiety	Decreased libido
Concentration/memory problems	Nausea, diarrhoea, constipation
Depressive or negative thinking (e.g. worthlessness, self-blame)	Menstrual disturbances
Poor self-confidence	
Alcohol, drug abuse	
Thoughts about death or suicide	

(Adapted from Kidman, 2006.)

Thinking changes in depression – your view of yourself and the world may seem very black. The depressed feelings worsen, with some describing depression as a black cloud, or like being in a dark tunnel with no light at the end. As a result, behaviour is affected, and you might, for example, become more withdrawn. Treatment for depression aims to give you tools to deal with negative thinking, feelings and behaviour, and break the **negative thinking and feeling cycle**.

Anxiety symptoms often occur in depression. These may include increased tension, headaches, muscle pain, restlessness and poor sleep. Panic attacks (sudden episodes of intense anxiety) may occur, or anxiety in social situations may worsen. If there is a tendency towards experiencing obsessive thoughts or behaviours, these too can worsen as a result of depression. Anxiety will be discussed in more detail later in this step.

Points to remember
- Understanding depression is important.
- Depression is common.
- In depression, mood is persistently and severely depressed, affecting the ability to cope and function.
- Depression is not weakness.
- It affects a person's thoughts, feelings and everyday functioning.
- Thinking changes in depression – there is a negative thinking and feeling cycle.
- Anxiety symptoms may occur or worsen.

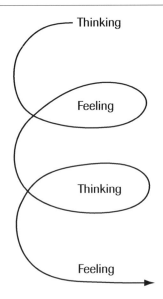

Thinking

Feeling

Thinking

Feeling

WHY DOES IT HAPPEN?

The cause of depression is not fully understood, but it is generally seen as a disorder that is made worse by life stress. The **'bio-psychosocial' model of depression** suggests that the causation of depression is related to biological, psychological and social factors (Engel, 1980).

1. Biological factors

➤ *Genetic*: depression can run in families: that is, there may be an inherited tendency to develop the disorder (Sadock and Sadock, 2007).

➤ *Neurotransmitter theory*: this theory suggests that there may be a change in levels of certain nerve messenger chemicals or neurotransmitters (serotonin, noradrenaline and dopamine) in the brain in depression (Sadock and Sadock, 2007). It is not clear whether these changes *cause* the depression, or are a *result* of the low mood.

➤ *Physical illness or medications*: infections such as glandular fever, or anaemia, low thyroid function or diabetes can produce symptoms of depression. An individual may be more prone to low mood at times of hormonal changes, such as menopause. Some prescribed medications have depression as a side effect, and drug abuse can be associated. That is why this program includes a medical review or check-up (*see* Step 2).

2. Psychological and social factors

➤ *Stressful life events*: stressful life events may have a role in the onset or relapse of depression.

　　1. Stress from personal tragedies, relationship breakdown or unemployment, for example, can contribute to depression.

　　2. **Loss and grief** may be a trigger (New Zealand National Health Committee, 1996).

3. Depression occurs more commonly at certain stages of life, such as adolescence, middle age, retirement age and in the elderly.
4. Traumatic early life experiences can be associated with later depression.

➤ *Personality*: an individual's personality may be a factor in depression. Some people have a tendency to be pessimistic and view things negatively, or be prone to worry. Early life traumas may influence personality and vulnerability to depression (Evans, Burrows and Norman, 2000).
➤ *Social issues*: lack of social support is a risk factor for depression. Social and economic factors can put a lot of stress on people, and decrease opportunities to look after health and well-being (Preston, 2004).

These factors may interact to trigger depression; for example, someone may have a family history of depression, and at a time of life stress may become depressed. It is important to recognise that **the individual is not to blame for the depression.**

RISK FACTORS	PROTECTIVE FACTORS
Social disadvantage	Close, positive personal relationships and social support
Family discord	
Poor social networks	Good family relationships
Parental mental illness	Supportive networks of friends
Child abuse	Achievements through study or sport
Difficult life events	Relaxed personality
Prior history of depression	Positive outlook on life
Being a female adolescent	Good coping strategies (e.g. stress management)
Anxiety	
Substance misuse	
Negative responses to stress	
Negative thinking	

(Adapted from Evans, Burrows and Norman, 2000; Preston, 2004.)

This table highlights that **there are risk factors as well as protective factors**. Some risk factors are hard to avoid, but others can be worked on. **It is important to be aware of the risk factors and try to minimise them,** just as you would with risk factors in, say, heart disease (Fava, Ruini and Mangelli, 2001). This program aims to help you reduce risk factors and to **develop the protective factors**.

WHAT ARE THE RISKS FROM DEPRESSION ITSELF?

Suicide is a real risk. Monitoring mood and treating depression adequately is therefore vitally important. Talk to family or friends, or to your GP or MHP, if you ever have suicidal thoughts. It is often a relief to share these troublesome thoughts with someone you trust.

Relationship breakdown is another serious consequence. It is important for family and friends to understand depression. Talking about the depression together or with a GP or MHP may be very helpful. Relationship counselling may be part of coping with the depression.

There is also a link between **alcohol use** and depression. Some people try and deal with the anxious or depressed feelings by drinking or **smoking** more, or using illicit drugs (Beyondblue, 2007).

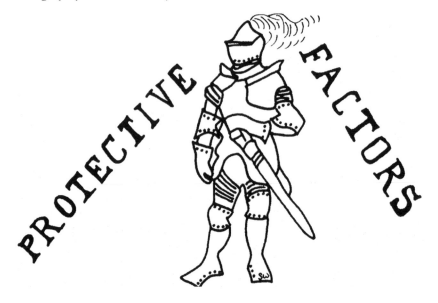

Points to remember
- There may be biological, psychological and social factors involved in depression.
- Stressful life events and loss and grief may be triggers of depression.
- The individual is not to blame for the depression.
- There are risk factors for depression as well as protective factors. It is important to be aware of the risk factors and to try and minimise them, and to develop the protective factors.
- There are risks from depression, including suicide, relationship breakdown, drug use.

WHY TREAT DEPRESSION?

Without treatment, depression often lasts for many months. Though you can endure the depression without getting treatment, it is often tough on you and your family. Most people find that getting help reduces the amount of distress they suffer from this painful problem.

With treatment you feel better sooner, and early treatment may help to keep the depression from becoming more severe. Treatment helps reduce the risks of depression, and also the risk of recurrence (Agency for Health Care Policy and Research, 1993; Ellis and The Royal Australian and New Zealand College of Psychiatrists Clinical Practice Team for Depression, 2004).

HOW IS DEPRESSION TREATED?

➤ **Effective treatments for depression are available**. Most commonly, treatment is provided by GPs (Pirkis, Stokes, Morley, *et al.*, 2006). The first step is establishing a trusting and reassuring relationship with your doctor or therapist (Ellis and The Royal Australian and New Zealand College of Psychiatrists Clinical Practice Team for Depression, 2004).

➤ Careful assessment of the individual is important. It is just as important in depression as in other conditions (such as diabetes or heart disease) to periodically assess how you are feeling and functioning, and to monitor your progress (Hickie, 2002).

➤ Treatment planning begins with setting goals towards recovery and staying well (*see* Step 2).

➤ Another early and ongoing treatment focus is **education** or providing information – about recovery from depression and the prevention of relapse.

➤ You will have **different priorities at different stages in your recovery**. For example, lifting low mood and dealing with sleep problems may be early concerns, and difficulties concentrating or dealing with anxiety may be later concerns. Keep talking with your GP or MHP, learning and working on your treatment goals.

➤ Treatment of depression addresses:
  - biological factors – through a more healthy lifestyle and possible use of medication
  - psychological and social factors – through psychotherapy or the talking therapies, along with practical coping strategies
  - it may also be important for individuals to address **spiritual** aspects of their lives.

➤ Remember that you *will* improve and that there *is* light at the end of the tunnel.

➤ **A range of treatment strategies is needed** to tackle depression, and treatment will vary from person to person because the effects of depression differ between people. You are an individual and this treatment program will be tailored to suit you.

➤ The individual with depression and their doctor are both guided in their choice of treatment by **severity of the depression**.
  - In *mild depression*, support and talking through problems and lifestyle changes are recommended (Ellis and Smith, 2002).
  - For *moderate to severe depression*, which impairs ability to function socially or at work, a combination of medication and psychotherapy (or talking therapy) is often used.

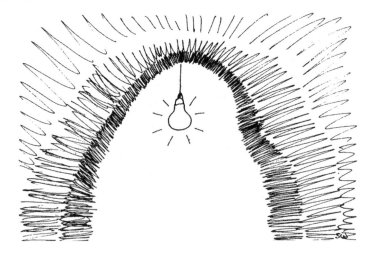

- Sometimes, medication is used as a first step in treatment, and is followed by psychotherapy, because it is often helpful to first lift the depression with medication, so that there is sufficient concentration and energy to talk about the psychological issues.
- Cognitive-behavioural therapy (CBT) has been found to be particularly effective in the treatment of mild to moderate depression, and in the prevention of relapses (Fava, Rafanelli, Grandi, *et al.*, 1998; Gloaguen, Cottraux, Cucherat, *et al.*, 1998).
- *Severe depression* may require hospitalisation. Feeling suicidal is a risk, and the individual should receive urgent help from their GP or MHP, or local crisis services if need be (WHO, 1997).

➤ Treatment will vary depending upon the stage of recovery from depression.
  - There is the **acute** or initial treatment stage, which aims to stabilise and relieve symptoms.
  - Next is a stage of **continuation** of treatment to prevent return of acute symptoms.
  - This is followed by a **maintenance** phase of treatment to help prevent relapse; the length of this phase depends on the history of the depression and the risk of developing a new episode (New Zealand National Health Committee, 1996).

➤ Regular follow-up is important in depression (Ellis and The Royal Australian and New Zealand College of Psychiatrists Clinical Practice Team for Depression, 2004).

Understanding and using antidepressant medication
➤ Antidepressants were developed in the 1950s and a large number of newer antidepressants are now available.
➤ Antidepressants are helpful when the following exist:
  - significant depression

- a previous positive response to medication
- a poor response to talking therapies
- more than one of the physical changes of depression (for example, altered sleep or low energy)
- agitation or worsening of panic
- suicidal ideas (Williams, 2000).

➤ Your GP can discuss the various types of antidepressants with you. There are several different classes of medication which work in different ways.

Points to remember
- Treatment of depression is effective. It reduces risks of depression and of relapse.
- You will improve.
- Ongoing monitoring of progress is important.
- There is a range of treatment strategies addressing the bio-psychosocial needs of the individual.
- Treatment varies depending upon the severity and stage of the depression.

One of the most frequently used classes of antidepressants is **SSRIs (selective serotonin reuptake inhibitors)**. These include:
- fluoxetine or 'Prozac', 'Lovan'
- paroxetine or 'Aropax'
- sertraline or 'Zoloft'
- fluvoxamine or 'Luvox'
- citalopram or 'Cipramil'
- escitalopram or 'Lexapro'.

SSRIs tend to be much better tolerated than the older types of antidepressants.
   Note – other newer antidepressants include:
- venlafaxine or 'Efexor'
- mirtazapine or 'Avanza'
- reboxetine or 'Edronax'.

If one antidepressant is found not to work well enough, your doctor may discuss swapping from one to another, or using other medications which can help stabilise mood.

➤ **Choice of antidepressant** depends on the individual person and the characteristics of the depression. Your doctor may recommend an SSRI or one of the other types of medication. **Sometimes several different antidepressants have to be tried** before the best one is found. There are national guidelines for managing depression that provide recommendations about antidepressant use (Australian and New Zealand College of Psychiatrists Clinical Practice Team for Depression, 2004).

➤ Antidepressants usually take several weeks to work, and may take up to six weeks to have a good effect. It is important to take the tablets regularly and for long enough to give them a good chance of working for you (Braddon J, Edwards S, Warrick T, *et al.*, 2007).

➤ Antidepressants have been found to be effective in many instances (Casacalenda, 2002), but are generally not advised for young people, and expert opinion should be sought.

➤ Like other medications, antidepressants can potentially have **side effects.** SSRIs, for example, may cause sleepiness, nausea, dry mouth and headache. There can be effects on sexual drive or functioning. Side effects often lessen over the first few weeks, so it is **definitely worth persevering**. Talk with your doctor if you have any queries about side effects.

➤ Unless the depression is severe, it is best to **'start low and go slow'** with antidepressants. This helps avoid unwanted side effects. Your GP can advise you on how to start on a low dose and gradually build up to the desired dose.

➤ There are recommended antidepressant doses, but remember, **dose depends on the individual and their response to treatment. Do not take a higher dose than your GP prescribes.** Talk about the dose with your doctor if you think a change is needed.

➤ It is **important to get into a regular routine** of taking antidepressants. You might place the medication somewhere where you will see it or write yourself a reminder note. *[Always keep medication out of the reach of children]*.

➤ Your GP will advise you on **how long** you will need to take the medication. It may be recommended that medication is taken for 6 to 12 months after the initial symptoms are lifted, or for longer in cases of recurrent depression (Ellis and Smith, 2002; Hickie, 2002).

➤ When stopping antidepressants it is best to gradually reduce them in the same way as they were gradually started. Antidepressants are not sedatives – **they are not addictive.** However, there may be side effects if the dose is suddenly reduced. Talk with your doctor first and work out a reduction plan.

➤ **Please do not stop taking the antidepressants without talking with your GP**. It is tempting to stop when you feel better, but the symptoms of depression tend to return quickly if medication is stopped too early. It is important to take the medication for the recommended length of time to get the best long-term effect, just as with antibiotics.

➤ If you need to use another type of medication (even a cold and flu tablet) while you are taking antidepressants it is important to check with your GP or pharmacist first. Antidepressants interact with some medications. This includes complementary medicines such as St John's Wort, which has an additive effect with antidepressants and can cause troublesome side effects (Braddon J, Edwards S, Warrick T, *et al.*, 2007).

➤ Try not to drink **alcohol**, or at least have a smaller amount, because it tends to aggravate depression, and also because antidepressants can interact with alcohol. Be careful, especially with driving.

➤ If you have any questions or concerns at any stage, speak with your GP. Your GP can seek the advice of a psychiatrist if need be.

(Based on Braddon J, Edwards S, Warrick T, *et al.*, 2007; Therapeutic Guidelines Limited, 2008.)

Points to remember
- Antidepressants are helpful in significant depression, especially if there are suicidal ideas.
- One of the most frequently used types is SSRIs.
- Choice of antidepressant and dose depends on the individual.
- Antidepressants take time to work.
- They are effective.
- They can have side effects, but these often lessen over time.
- PERSISTENCE is important.
- Please don't stop taking antidepressants without talking with your GP.

Psychotherapy or the talking therapies and depression

There are a number of **talking therapies** for depression. They aim to help the person understand what is happening. Doctors and other health professionals draw on a range of approaches, including:
- counselling
- problem-solving therapy
- cognitive-behavioural psychotherapy
- acceptance and commitment therapy
- interpersonal psychotherapy
- insight-oriented psychotherapy
- other therapies (Evans, Burrows and Norman, 2000).

➤ The term **counselling** covers a wide range of techniques. The main focus is on providing non-judgemental support that allows people to talk over their problems. Having support during a very difficult time is really important (WHO, 1997).

➤ **Problem-solving therapy** provides techniques for a person to address problems in life so that the problems become less overwhelming. This therapy has been shown to be effective in depression (Huibers, Beurskens, Bleijenberg, *et al.*, 2003).

➤ **Cognitive-behavioural therapy** (CBT) is one way of helping people to cope with depression, stress or anxiety. It is based on the idea that our thinking and behaviours influence how we feel. CBT teaches the individual to be aware of and challenge negative thoughts that produce fear (anxiety). It also includes techniques that facilitate behaviour change. In doing so, it helps tackle the symptoms of anxiety and depression.

➤ CBT involves a lot more than just 'positive thinking'. It involves learning more helpful thinking patterns. It has been shown to be effective in treating depression and preventing relapse (Gloaguen, Cottraux, Cucherat, *et al.*, 1998). A range of CBT skills will be taught during this treatment program (*see* Steps 4 and 5).

➤ **Acceptance and commitment therapy (ACT)** is a 'mindfulness-based behaviour therapy', which incorporates mindfulness, i.e. experiencing the present moment (Segal, Williams and Teasdale, 2002), and 'values-guided behavioural strategies' (Harris, 2007). Mindfulness and ACT are further explained in Step 5.

➤ **Interpersonal psychotherapy (IPT)** focuses on the impact of relationship difficulties on the depression; mood and interpersonal events are seen as dependent on each other. IPT may involve working through feelings of grief or conflict, or difficulties relating to people socially, for example, by teaching assertiveness (Davies, 2000).

➤ **Insight-oriented psychotherapy** aims to assist the person in understanding possible psychological causes of their depression (Evans, Burrows and Norman, 2000).

➤ There are other types of psychotherapy and different therapists may have a preference for using one over another, depending on their training.

   • One that you may hear about is **narrative therapy**. This form of therapy involves the therapist and the individual patient working together to identify what the individual wants in their own life, and how to utilise their own knowledge and skills (White and Denborough, 1998).

   • **Well-being therapy** focuses on well-being rather than relieving symptoms of illness and aims to increase personal effectiveness (Fava, Rafanelli, Cazzaro, *et al.*, 1998).

GPs or MHPs may choose to use a combination of talking therapies, and **this program also incorporates useful aspects of a number of different talking therapies.**

   GPs tend to be what is called **eclectic or multimodal** in their approach – that is, they draw on a range of treatment approaches (Dryden and Mytton, 1999). This is because they are used to dealing with such a wide range of problems and issues in their practice.

Other aspects of treatment

➤ You will remember that depression affects ability to cope and function on a day-to-day basis. This treatment program aims to help you with **overall functioning**.

➤ Treatment also focuses on your overall **well-being** (Koppe, 2002). It highlights the importance of healthy lifestyle, and tackling problem areas such as managing stress, sleep difficulties, or getting more involved socially.

➤ Some depression is seasonal and related to the amount of daylight. Talk with your GP if you think this is a factor, as treatment may be assisted with a light box.

➤ You may also want to talk about natural or **complementary therapies** with your GP if you have a particular interest in this area. Some useful references have been listed under Resources at Step 10.

HOW MY GP OR MHP CAN HELP

➤ Your GP can help you manage the depression by providing **information and advice** about treatment. Having assessed how severe the depression is, they can discuss with you whether antidepressant medication is recommended.

➤ Your GP will assess your physical health, provide lifestyle advice and help monitor your progress.

➤ The aim of this treatment program is to provide a **holistic approach** to managing the depression. Your GP or MHP will guide you through the program, but you have the responsibility of putting the program into practice.

➤ Your GP or MHP will discuss how you are feeling and review any problems you may be having. Together you can discuss any concerns about treatment and consider whether any changes are needed.

➤ Each time you go to see your GP or MHP, it is helpful to **write down how you have been feeling and any questions** that you want to discuss. You could use the notes page at the end of each step, or your journal.

➤ Another hint is to mention main concerns at the beginning of your appointment, so they definitely get addressed.

➤ Don't worry about what the doctor may be thinking – any question or concern is important and worth bringing up. Write down information from your discussions to aid remembering, especially in the early stages of depression.

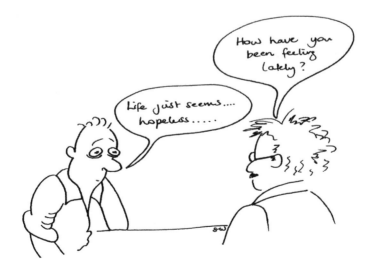

HOW CAN I HELP MYSELF?

➤ It is helpful to **gather information** about depression and try and understand it as much as possible. **Talking** with family or friends can be very helpful – especially for the support they can give. Your GP or MHP can talk with them and you together if you wish, to answer any questions about depression or its treatment.

➤ Visiting the local library or bookshop for extra resources can be useful, and occasionally there are very good programs on the radio or television about depression or anxiety.

➤ Utilise internet resources (*see* Step 10).

➤ It is suggested that you **be honest** with your family and your doctor about how you are feeling – only you know how you are feeling and what your concerns are. Expressing what you think and feel is part of the recovery and healing process. It is important **not to keep things to yourself – work on sharing your feelings and concerns and have a cry if need be.**

➤ No questions or concerns are too small to raise with your GP or MHP. Some people fear that their question will be thought of as silly – this is not the case. **Write down** your questions as you become aware of them. You could use your journal or the notes page at the end of each section. It can be very frustrating to get into the doctor's office and not be able to remember that important question.

➤ Some people find it really helpful to **attend a support group to talk with others** who are experiencing the same sort of problems. It can be really useful to attend a group and see that you are **not alone** in dealing with depression, and to share ideas. Speak with your GP or MHP or check with your local Community Health Centre about what is available in your area.

➤ **Working through this treatment program is a very positive step**. It has been designed with the aim of helping you to recover and look after yourself in the future, by focusing on support, strategies and skills.

➤ You will also find **your own positive ways to help yourself**. You are the expert on yourself and will think of things that will help you as an individual. There may have been things that you have done in the past that helped you to recover from an episode of depression, or deal with another illness or a crisis.

➤ Along with this treatment guide, it is suggested that you use an exercise book:
  • to jot down ideas that you have, or points that come out of discussions with your GP, MHP, family and friends, or your reading
  • to use as a reflective journal to record how you are feeling, what you have been thinking about or what you have been doing. Some people prefer to write poetry or draw to express themselves
  • to use more as a scrapbook for collecting useful and meaningful articles, pictures or sayings.

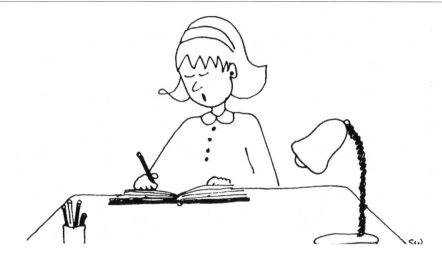

➤ One of the things that this program emphasises is **self-care.** This is **part of a holistic approach** to managing the depression. Strategies for coping with stress and sleep difficulties will be looked at. When you are stressed or feeling down, it can be tempting to increase the use of alcohol and cigarettes as a way of trying to cope. But for your health and well-being it is important to avoid overusing alcohol or cigarettes. The same applies to the use of illicit drugs. Sleeping tablets may be needed in the first week or two, but it is best to avoid relying on these in the longer term.

➤ Later in the program, Step 3 looks at healthy lifestyle issues. You may need to gradually change some aspects of your lifestyle, such as more healthy eating or exercising. Step 7 is all about becoming more active. So begin to think about the **activities** that you have enjoyed in the past, as part of the recovery process is gradually re-engaging in these sorts of activities.

➤ The KBA program is designed to run over 12 months, incorporating all the phases of treatment (acute, continuation and maintenance). It is important, however, to keep referring back to what you have learned after the 12 months has passed, and to **keep the strategies and skills going.**

➤ See your GP or MHP regularly for follow-up during the 12 months. The whole purpose of all your work and effort right now is to keep you well in the future.

WHAT FAMILY AND FRIENDS CAN DO

Depression can be difficult for family and friends to understand. They may be confused and concerned, as often the depressed person withdraws from them or is irritable. Providing them with information about depression or taking them to an appointment with your GP or MHP can be very helpful.

They need to have an understanding of the nature of depression and be aware that recovery takes time. Be honest with family and friends whom you choose to confide in about the depression and how you feel. As you recover, try to become more involved with people again.

A useful reference book for family and friends is Golant and Golant's *What to Do When Someone You Love is Depressed: a practical, compassionate, and helpful guide*. Websites like the beyondblue site (www.beyondblue.org.au) can be very helpful. See further books and websites under Resources in Step 10.

Points to remember
- There is a range of talking therapies for depression, including counselling, cognitive-behavioural therapy (CBT), interpersonal therapy (IPT) and acceptance commitment therapy (ACT).
- This program for depression treatment and relapse prevention incorporates aspects of a number of different talking therapies.
- It aims to help you with overall functioning and well-being, by using a holistic approach.
- Work with your GP or MHP – they can provide information and advice, support and counselling/therapy.
- Gather information; write down your questions.
- Talk with family and friends.
- Be honest with your family and doctor.
- You are not alone in dealing with the depression.
- Working through this program is a positive step.
- The program focuses on self-care.
- Find your own ways to help yourself.
- Think about keeping a journal.
- Keep the newly-learned skills going in the future.

WHAT TO EXPECT IN THE EARLY AND LATER STAGES OF RECOVERY

Remember the discussion about the **three phases in the treatment** of depression – **acute, continuation and maintenance** (New Zealand National Health Committee, 1996).

The acute or early stages of treatment are directed towards assessment and to starting the appropriate treatment so that you begin to feel less unwell. If treatment involves antidepressants, these **take time to work**. Often, individuals notice an improvement in their mood at two to three weeks, but an effect may not be noticed for up to six weeks.

Whatever the treatment, whether medication or talking, it is **important that you keep going with it.** Recovery involves learning new skills and strategies, and these take time and practice. Through this program you have made a **commitment** to help yourself. Always remember that you *will* improve and that there *is* hope.

It is tempting, as you feel better, to stop taking medication, stop looking after yourself, or revert to unhelpful or negative ways of thinking or behaving. **Maintain the skills and strategies** that you learn, and keep looking after your emotional and physical well- being.

WHAT IS RELAPSE OR RECURRENCE OF DEPRESSION, AND WHEN AM I AT RISK?

Relapse and recurrence of depression have very similar meanings. Relapse of depression means that there is an early return of symptoms, before full recovery. Recurrence of depression refers to return of symptoms after a time of being symptom-free (Kupfer, 1991). Don't get too concerned about the difference, as we tend to use the words interchangeably in practice.

The graph below illustrates relapse and recurrence of depression:

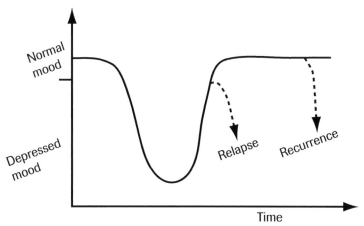

(Adapted from Kupfer, 1991.)

Unfortunately depression can be a recurrent illness. It is viewed as a chronic type of illness, with periods of wellness and periods of recurrence. In the primary care setting depression is reported to recur in about 40% of individuals. That is why this treatment program has been devised. It aims to help you to get well and stay well in the future.

However, **it is important to maintain a sense of hope and perspective**. Many people remain well and do not relapse (Van Weel-Baumgarten, 1998).

WHAT ABOUT ANXIETY?

People often experience symptoms of depression and anxiety at the same time. Many of the symptoms are similar, and can interfere with daily functioning. It can be difficult at times to work out which is the main problem. Sometimes a person may have an anxiety disorder and then develop depression. Or depression itself can trigger symptoms of anxiety.

Anxiety is similar to fear, but it occurs in the absence of a specific danger. It is usually in response to *anticipated* problems, rather than *actual* problems. Some people can feel constantly anxious. Episodes of extreme fear or panic, known as panic episodes, may be experienced (Bloch and Singh, 1997).

The diagram below shows the **overlap between symptoms** of anxiety and depression.

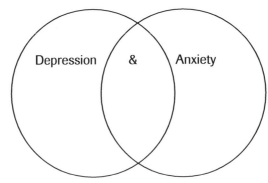

(Adapted from Evans, Burrows and Norman, 2000.)

It is important to identify and treat an underlying depression, and it is also important to deal with the anxiety symptoms. This program includes **strategies to help reduce symptoms of anxiety,** including stress management and relaxation techniques and helpful thinking or cognitive strategies (*see* Steps 3–5). Some antidepressant medication helps reduce the symptoms of anxiety as well as treating the depression.

For reference the anxiety disorders include:

➤ generalised anxiety – prolonged and excessive worry
➤ panic disorder – sudden episodes of overwhelming fear – may be associated with agoraphobia (fear in settings where escape is difficult or help is not available)
➤ specific phobias – excessive fear of a definable object (such as spiders or heights)
➤ social anxiety – excessive fear of embarrassment in social situations
➤ obsessive-compulsive disorder – repetitive thoughts and fears and compulsive behaviours
➤ post-traumatic stress disorder – following an event that is extremely traumatic.

(Based on American Psychiatric Association, 2000.)

You may be familiar with some of these or want to talk more about them with your GP or MHP.

Points to remember
- Treatment takes time; it is important to persist.
- Relapse and recurrence refer to return of the symptoms of depression.
- Symptoms of anxiety and depression may be experienced at the same time.
- This treatment program involves strategies to help reduce anxiety.

NOTES PAGE

Assessment and goal setting

'The journey of a thousand miles begins with one step' (Lao Tzu)

A MEDICAL REVIEW OR CHECK-UP

A number of physical illnesses can be linked to depression. These include diabetes, heart problems, hypothyroidism (low thyroid function), vitamin deficiency (Vitamin B12 and folate), and nervous system conditions such as Parkinson's disease. It is possible for some medications (such as anti-high blood pressure medications or the contraceptive pill) to trigger depression (Sadock and Sadock, 2007).

Your GP will ensure that any medical condition that might be a cause of depression has been ruled out, or is identified and addressed. The medications that you are taking will also be checked. Together you will work out which medications best control your health problems and have the least adverse effect on your mood. It is also important to check that any other medical problems you have are well controlled so that you feel as physically well as possible.

REVIEW OF THE PSYCHOSOCIAL ASSESSMENTS

Your GP or MHP may have given you a questionnaire to help assess your mood and how well you have been managing on a day-to-day basis. Discuss the results together – this will help you understand how the depression or any associated anxieties are affecting you. You might want to write down in your journal, or on the notes page at the end of this step, any thoughts or ideas that stem from the assessments. The assessments will help you and your doctor plan your treatment together.

GOAL SETTING

It is helpful to have a sense of direction in managing the depression. One way of doing this is to consider the sort of things you value in life (Harris, 2007). We all have values in relation to key areas in life such as family and relationships, our health, work or education, leisure activities, community life, the environment or spirituality. Work with your GP or MHP to establish a number of goals directed towards coping and recovery. You may choose to work on a particular key area to begin with, such as health. Over time it is important to choose goals that fit with what you value in life.

A goal is an aim or want – it is about where you want to be. It may help to ask yourself 'what would I like to happen?' Your GP or MHP will guide you through the following **three steps of goal setting.** (Adapted from Kidman, 2006; World Health Organization Collaborating Centre for Mental Health and Substance Abuse, 2000.)

1. **Make a list of what you see as your short-term goals right now.**
   - **Goals need to be realistic,** as it is best to set a goal that can be achieved. Any goals you have, no matter how small, are important.
   - **Be specific** about what you want.
   - How you define 'short-term' will vary for different people at the different stages of recovery. You may make a goal for **an hour, a day, a week or a month**.
   - It is best that goals be written in the **positive sense**, about what you *will* do rather than what you *don't want* to do.
   - Choose goals that are not dependent on other people; that is, choose **independent** goals.

Here are some examples of goals.

Over the next week:
➤ to get up and dressed each day
➤ to go on one outing.

Over the next three months:
➤ to find time to do some exercise
➤ to learn how to deal with negative thoughts.

Discuss how to write your goals with your GP or MHP.

SHORT-TERM GOALS
1.
2.
3.
4.

2. **Prioritise or rank the goals according to their importance to you right now.**

PRIORITISE YOUR GOALS

1.

2.

3.

4.

---

3. **Now break down one important goal into a number of *steps* that help you achieve this goal.** The steps need to be as small and specific and achievable as possible ('baby steps' are the most achievable). Also, identify any help that you might need to achieve your goals.

An example of breaking a goal down into steps.
The goal, 'to find time to do some exercise', could be broken down into the following steps.
   1. Think about how a small amount of exercise could be incorporated into the week.
   2. Start with a walk once a week.
   3. Increase the number of walks each week.

STEPS TO ACHIEVE MY 'NUMBER 1' PRIORITY GOAL

1.

2.

3.

4.

I plan to achieve this goal by: _____(date)
I will know that I have achieved it because:

Repeat Step 3 with your other goals:

STEPS TO ACHIEVE MY GOAL

1.

2.

3.

4.

I plan to achieve this goal by: _____(date)
I will know that I have achieved it because:

STEPS TO ACHIEVE MY GOAL

1.

2.

3.

4.

I plan to achieve this goal by: _____(date)
I will know that I have achieved it because:

STEPS TO ACHIEVE MY GOAL

1.

2.

3.

4.

I plan to achieve this goal by: _____(date)
I will know that I have achieved it because:

It is important to **review and rewrite your goal lists regularly**. They may change as different aspects of recovery assume more importance. For example, improving your health may be a priority at one time; resuming an interest or returning to work at another. As you feel able, you can focus on **longer-term goals.**

A spare sheet with all three tables on it is provided in this step. You can make copies when you want to rewrite or add new goals.

MONITORING YOUR PROGRESS

It is useful to monitor your mood by using a scale from 0 to 10 to rate the depression, where 0 means no depression and 10 the most severe depression. This will help you and your GP or MHP monitor changes in your mood and your progress over time.

Review your progress regularly. Did you achieve your goal? If you did, well done! Enjoy your sense of achievement and make sure you acknowledge your success. For example, you might have a coffee with a friend to celebrate. Then, set a slightly harder goal for next time.

Talk with your GP or MHP regularly about your goals. Did you miss your goal? If you did, that's okay. You will probably find that you made some progress toward achieving your goal. Try to see this as an opportunity to celebrate the progress that you did make. Also, you can plan how to better achieve the goal next time. Perhaps you need to break the goal down into smaller ones, or add some more steps. Don't give up. You can do it!

A sheet to photocopy when you want to review your goals:

LIST OF SHORT-TERM GOALS

1.

2.

3.

4.

PRIORITISE YOUR GOALS

1.

2.

3.

4.

STEPS TO ACHIEVE MY PRIORITY GOAL

1.

2.

3.

4.

I plan to achieve this goal by: _____(date)

I will know that I have achieved it because:

Points to remember
- Work on goals that are of value or important to you.
- Initially focus on short-term goals.
- Goals need to be realistic, positive and not dependent on others.
- Prioritise your goals.
- Break goals down into small, specific and achievable steps.
- Review and rewrite your goal lists regularly.

NOTES PAGE

Healthy lifestyle issues

How can I help myself?

Think about the term 'lifestyle' and what it means to you. You might want to jot down your ideas here.

_____

_____

_____

One definition relates to the way in which we live. Every day we eat and sleep, and carry out a range of activities. These may relate to simply existing and meeting basic human needs, or may relate to work, family duties or leisure.

One of the questions asked during Step 1 was 'How can I help myself?' Self-care, or taking care of yourself, is very important. This involves looking after every aspect of yourself – whether physical, emotional, social, vocational (work-related) or spiritual. These areas are all inter-related. That's why it is important not to ignore your physical health, for example, when feeling down.

Whatever the cause of your depression, the depression itself tends to indicate that some changes in lifestyle are needed. What follows is a discussion about healthy lifestyle changes that may help (Stern, 1998).

How can you make self-care a greater part of your lifestyle? Jot down three or four ways in which you might do this.

_____

_____

_____

_____

Now let's look at some of the ways to take care of yourself, and in doing so, improve the depression.

HEALTHY EATING

This section is about eating healthily. The word *diet* in the term 'healthy diet' does not refer to reducing food intake to lose weight. It refers to what we eat to maintain our health and well-being.

When feeling depressed it is common to lose your appetite or to eat more than is needed for comfort. But eating a healthy diet can help us feel better physically and mentally. The saying, 'you are what you eat', has a lot of truth in it. Think about times when you have eaten well. Did you feel better in yourself?

If a friend asked you 'What is a healthy diet?' what would your answer be?

_____

_____

_____

_____

_____

_____

You would probably apply commonsense, and this is a good approach.

The Australian Dietary Guidelines suggest that healthy diets should:
➤ *provide all essential nutrients in adequate amounts required for good health*
➤ *avoid excess nutrients that might contribute to disease (e.g. excess fat or sugar)*
➤ *be enjoyable.*
(Department of Health and Ageing, 2005)

The Australian Dietary Guidelines have been produced to provide a guide to healthy eating. They include the following.
  a. Enjoy a wide variety of nutritious foods:
    • eat plenty of vegetables and fruits
    • eat plenty of cereals, preferably whole-grain, including breads, pasta and noodles
    • include lean meat, fish, poultry and alternatives such as legumes (e.g. soya beans, lentils) and nuts
    • include reduced-fat dairy foods
    • ensure that you drink enough water every day.
  b. Take care to:
    • eat fat in moderation and limit saturated fat
    • choose foods low in salt
    • limit alcohol intake if you choose to drink
    • eat only moderate amounts of sugars and foods containing added sugars.

It is important to prevent weight gain by being physically active and eating according to your needs (Department of Health and Ageing, 2005). To reduce saturated fat in the diet, we can eat foods such as fish, nuts, fruit and vegetables, olive oil or avocados, rather than foods such as margarine, ice cream or chocolate. It is good to choose low-fat dairy food and lean cuts of meat, and to use healthy cooking methods such as grilling.

A few other healthy eating ideas may be helpful.

➤ A commonsense guide is to choose and enjoy healthy foods when you are hungry, and stop eating when you sense that you have had enough. If you are eating a food containing a lot of sugar or fat, then have a little rather than a lot – moderation is the key. And even if your appetite is down, try to eat regularly.

➤ Some foods raise the blood sugar level higher than others. If we eat a lot of these foods we are more at risk of illnesses such as diabetes. Generally, we are better off eating what are called 'low G.I.' (glycaemic index) foods that raise sugar levels the least but give you sustained energy. These are the sort of foods already mentioned as healthy – such as whole-grain breads, pasta, noodles and legumes, unprocessed cereals and fruits (Brand-Miller, 2000).

➤ Research has shown that eating oily fish that is rich in fatty acids, such as sardines, tuna and salmon, is good for your health. Fish oils can help prevent heart disease and are also important in brain functioning (CSIRO, 2007). If you don't like to eat fish, fish-oil supplements are available.

➤ If an individual's diet is healthy, dietary supplements are generally not needed. However, you may find taking a multivitamin of some assistance, and some individuals find calcium and magnesium a useful preparation. Talk with your GP if you would like to discuss this issue further.

BECOMING MORE ACTIVE AND EXERCISING

Exercise has a positive effect on how you feel (Lawlor, 2001). It develops fitness, helps you relax and promotes a sense of well-being. When you exercise, brain chemicals called endorphins are released and help you feel good. Exercise during the day aids sleep at night.

What sort of exercise do you enjoy or have you enjoyed in the past?

_____

_____

_____

_____

Exercise includes walking, swimming, playing football, going to the gym and gardening. Even house cleaning and washing the car are exercise! Walking is a great form of exercise. Having a dog to walk gives you a reason to walk, and can be a very social activity, for example, by giving opportunities to chat with other dog owners at the park.

Walking on the beach or in the park, and enjoying nature while you walk, can be very peaceful. Some people enjoy yoga or tai chi, and again these are very relaxing.

Think now about how you can make time to exercise – making it part of your routine is helpful. For example, take the stairs at work instead of the lift. Jot down some ideas.

_____

_____

Try to make exercise part of your life. You may want to think about writing up exercise as a goal to help towards recovery and staying well. You can use the spare goal-setting sheet provided. The goal-setting principles explained earlier apply – choose straightforward and realistic goals. A first goal may be getting started!

A good guide is to start with a small amount of exercise. Always do some stretches beforehand, and slowly build up the amount of exercise you do. You will be surprised how your fitness improves.

SLEEPING BETTER

'Sleep is the common chain that ties health and our bodies together'

(Thomas Dekker)

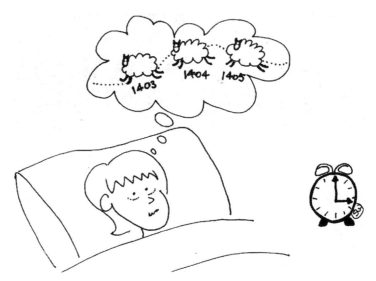

Sleep is part of our everyday life and functioning, and until it is a problem, we often take sleep for granted. Unfortunately sleep patterns can be upset in depression – it may be hard to get to sleep, or there may be a tendency to wake up in the early hours of the morning and have difficulty getting back to sleep. Some people with depression find they sleep too much. Sleep quality may be poor in depression.

Try not to worry about finding it difficult to sleep, as anxiety itself deters sleep. Even if you are not actually asleep, resting and relaxing is still beneficial to the mind and body.

Keeping a sleep diary may be a good place to start in working on your sleep. This involves keeping a record of the day, your activities and sleep patterns. Here is an example.

TIME OF DAY	ACTIVITY	SLEEP
7 p.m.	Dinner	
8 p.m.	TV	
9 p.m.		
10 p.m.		Nap in front of TV
11 p.m.		
12 midnight		Off to sleep
1 a.m.		
2 a.m.		Awake again

Keep the sleep diary for the full 24 hours, and keep it for at least a few days. You will then have a good amount of information to discuss with your GP. Here is a diary to copy and complete.

TIME OF DAY	ACTIVITY	SLEEP

Also, think about things that seem to help your sleep, and talk with your GP. Here are some other tips that can help you with sleep.

➤ Accept that your sleep will be disturbed for a while, but have the attitude that you will do the best you can. You may need to place fewer demands on yourself, and be careful with driving if you are fatigued.

➤ Accept that your sleep will improve over time.

➤ Aim to re-establish a sleep routine, that is, going to bed at about the same time each night, and getting up at the same time each morning (regardless of what your sleep has been like).

➤ Develop a bed-time ritual, for example – hot milk drink, teeth and toilet, then bed.

➤ Bed is a place for sleeping – not doing work or watching television.

➤ Have a wind-down or relaxation time before going to bed – think about what you would find relaxing. Enjoy a warm bath, but have this a good hour or two before bed. You might read for a while or listen to peaceful music but do this in another room. Then go to bed when you feel sleepy.

➤ Specific relaxation techniques can be helpful to assist you in going to sleep – these will be explained in Step 4.

➤ If you wake up during the night and are lying awake, first try not to let it worry you. Repeat your relaxation techniques. If you are still awake after 30 minutes then get up and repeat your wind-down.

➤ In general, if you are not sleeping well at night, avoid sleeping during the day, or dozing off in the chair at night. A day-time nap is fine if you are tired and managing to sleep at night.

➤ Managing stress, so that your mind is more peaceful when you go to bed, is important. Stress management will be discussed later in this step.

➤ If something is worrying you at night and there is nothing you can do about it, try writing it down so that you can deal with it the next day. Keep a pen and paper next to the bed.

➤ Make sure that your bed and pillow are comfortable, and the bedroom is at a comfortable temperature.

➤ Some people find that a couple of drops of an essential oil such as lavender, on the pillow, is soothing. *[General safeguards for aromatherapy are: always check first that you are not sensitive to the smell of the oil or allergic to it (by a patch test on the skin with the oil diluted in water); avoid contact with the eyes; do not use if pregnant. Essential oils are flammable, so avoid open flames.]*

➤ Exercising during the day means you will be more physically tired at night. Avoid exercising heavily before bed, as this tends to make you more alert.

➤ Avoid too much caffeine or alcohol – both can disturb sleep.

➤ Avoid overeating in the evening.

➤ On the other hand having a light supper (for example, a banana and milk drink) can aid sleep.

(Based on White, 1998; UK Royal College of Psychiatrists website; Rankin-Box, 2001.)

What about sleeping tablets?

Sometimes sleeping tablets are useful in the early or acute phase of depression. It is not advised to take these long-term because of potential problems. Some anti-depressant medications are more helpful for sleep than others. You may want to discuss sleep and medication further with your GP.

Points to remember
- Lifestyle refers to the way in which we live.
- Self-care is important.

- In depression, lifestyle changes may be needed and be helpful.
- When feeling depressed, appetite is often affected.
- A healthy diet provides all the nutrients needed, avoids excess, and is enjoyable.
- Exercise has a positive effect on how you feel.
- Try to make exercise part of your life – slowly build up the amount that you do.
- Sleep can be upset in depression. Try not to worry.
- Keep a sleep diary, and see the tips that can help you with sleep.

REDUCING STRESS
First – how to identify stress in your life

The first step in reducing stress is to identify what stress is and how it impacts on your life. We have all experienced stress and know what it feels like to be stressed. It is part of life, and happens in response to the demands in life. But it is still an individual experience, and has different meanings to different people. Some people might describe stress as tension, others as worry, or feeling overwhelmed or out of control.

What does stress mean to you and how does it interfere with your life?

_____
_____
_____
_____

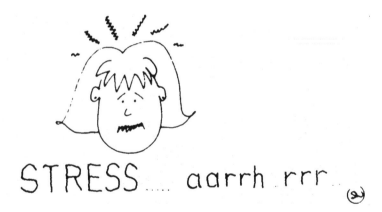

Stress can be triggered by many external factors, for example, significant life events such as injury, illness, relationship breakdown, or loss of a loved one through death. Everyday concerns, such as financial or work worries, or family problems, can trigger stress (Evans, Coman and Burrows, 1998).

The experience of stress is also influenced by internal factors. That is, how an individual responds to stress will be determined by their:

➤ perception of the stress (some people are threatened by giving a speech, others enjoy it)

➤ personality factors, including 'locus of control' (perceived degree of control over what happens)
➤ expectations of themselves (some people have very high expectations of how they will perform and feel stressed by wanting to achieve such a high level)
➤ coping skills (what useful skills have been learned in the past to help cope with stress)
➤ available support (Evans, Coman and Burrows, 1998).

Make a list of things that create stress in your life. Try to be specific, e.g. too much work, having difficulty coping in social situations.

_____
_____
_____
_____
_____
_____
_____
_____

How would you grade your level of stress right now on a scale of 0 to 10 (0 = no stress, and 10 = extreme stress)?

0 _____ 10

Stress is best seen as a process involving the following steps:
➤ a demand or pressure (called a stressor) is placed on the individual
➤ the mind and body react
➤ some response is shown.

For example, moving house is often a stressor. The individual reacts with thoughts and feelings ('I'll be glad when this is over'), may develop physical symptoms such as muscle tension, and responds in different ways – asking for help, doing lots of work!

The responses of the mind and body to stress are actually **adaptive,** that is, they help us to survive in dangerous situations. If you are crossing a busy road and a car is speeding towards you, the body will respond by producing a hormone in the body called adrenaline. This will get your heart pumping quickly to help you run to the side of the road. This is called the **'fight-or-flight' response** (Benson, 1977).

Stress can be both a positive and negative experience for the individual. Feeling stressed before an exam may push you to study hard and do well as a result. On the other hand, if your response to the stress is to avoid studying, you will probably not perform well. **Negative effects of stress,** especially prolonged stress, include the following.

PHYSICAL	EMOTIONAL	BEHAVIOURAL	SOCIAL
Headaches	Irritability	Changes in eating, smoking or alcohol use	Inability to fulfil social roles
Tiredness	Anger		
Sleeping problems	Decreased concentration		Impact on relationships at home or work
Muscle cramps		Nail biting	
Palpitations	Over-reaction	Decreased libido	
Chest pains	Symptoms of anxiety and depression		

(Evans, Coman, and Burrows, 1998)

A problem can arise if stress continues for some time. The body uses up a lot of energy trying to respond, and we can become exhausted and more prone to illness, such as infection.

The diagram below highlights the links between stress and physical as well as emotional well-being.

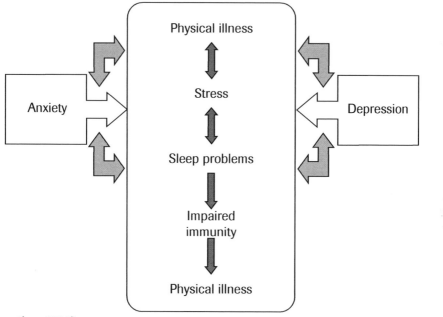

(Wheatley, 2000)

Second – what you can do about stress?

It is impossible to remove stress from life completely. It may be possible to reduce it, however, by managing it differently. This can be done by working on the external factors causing stress, or changing how you deal with it as an individual.

Think back to the list that you made of things creating stress in your life. Are there any situations causing stress that could be changed in some way? Write down what changes you would like and how you might bring about those changes.

_____
_____
_____
_____
_____

Are there any factors within yourself that you might work on to be better able to manage stress? Would it help to lower expectations of how you perform in certain situations, or would it help to learn how to relax? Jot down your thoughts.

_____
_____
_____
_____
_____

It is amazing what some individuals manage to cope with in their life. They may think they are not coping well, but have in fact coped with an enormous amount of stress, and have managed very well. It is worth looking at the different ways in which people cope.

There are two different types of strategies for coping with stress.

1. Problem-focused strategies – managing the problem causing the stress (used when we feel we have some control over what is happening) – include taking direct action. For example, we may make a plan to change or avoid the stressful situation, or to speak directly to a person who is making us feel stressed.
2. Emotion-focused strategies – managing the emotional response to the problem causing the stress (used when we feel the stress is outside our immediate control) – include putting aside the problem, blaming oneself, getting emotional support from friends or withdrawing (Evans, Coman and Burrows, 1998).

Do you respond in the same way when stressed by different things?

_____
_____
_____
_____
_____

What **coping strategies** do you generally use?

_____
_____
_____
_____
_____

Do you think that these are effective or ineffective?

_____
_____
_____
_____
_____
_____
_____
_____

It can be helpful to think about what the main concern is underlying the feeling of stress. If the main concern is feeling overwhelmed, then ask yourself whether there is too much work or if more help is needed? Is the stress about being tired – would rest or being more physically fit help? Is it about procrastinating and needing to learn how to get on with things? Maybe it is about needing to be more confident or assertive, or maybe thinking more positively would help.

(**Note** – dealing with procrastination, developing self-confidence and assertiveness, along with positive thinking, are all covered in Steps 4–8)

In relation to the things that are causing you stress, what can you identify as your main concerns?

_____
_____
_____
_____
_____
_____
_____

Can you think of any other strategies that might help you deal with these concerns? Examples might be taking a break from work or learning how to relax.

_____
_____
_____
_____
_____
_____
_____

(**Note** – The role of thinking in stress and anxiety will be discussed in Step 5. A range of relaxation techniques will be explained in Step 4.)

What about work-related stress? This is a common problem with the pressures of the workplace (Evans and Wagon, 2002). The stress may be related to work volume, fear of losing the job, or interpersonal relationships. Or it may be related to internal factors such as placing high expectations on yourself.

Have a think about what aspects of your work are causing you stress and talk about them with your GP. It can be very helpful to apply the problem-solving technique outlined in Step 4 to work-related problems. Don't forget that small changes, such as taking breaks, can really help you cope with a day at work.

For general stress don't forget **general measures** such as the following.

➤ Keep your **mind and body** as **healthy** as possible. This helps create more resilience when you have to deal with stress. (Refer back to the earlier discussion on healthy eating and sleeping better.)

➤ Many people find **exercise** is a good way to relieve stress. Walking is a cheap and pleasant form of exercise. Simply stretching the body can help too. Paul Wilson, who has written a series of books about being 'Calm', describes a stretching exercise called the 'windmill' which helps relieve stress. [Note – *only do stretches that you feel that you can manage physically.*]

The windmill involves the following steps.

---

1. In the standing position, bend the knees slightly. Bend the elbows and cross the wrists about navel level. Your palms should face upwards.
2. Move your arms upwards in a big circle, breathing in and straightening your legs as you do so.
3. Complete the circle, exhale and let your knees bend again.
4. Repeat these steps a number of times.
5. Then reverse the movement several times.
6. Move slowly and smoothly. Relax!

(Wilson, 1995)

➤ It may help to reduce drinks containing the stimulant caffeine, such as coffee and some cola drinks, which can have effects on the body similar to those created in stressful situations. Moderation is a good approach.

➤ On the other hand, a cup of tea at a stressful time can be helpful. And some herbal teas are reported to be calming.

➤ Slow down – **avoid hurrying**. This may involve not overloading yourself. Work out what commitments and workload you can manage. Know what your limits are especially when feeling anxious or depressed. You may need to think about what you expect of yourself, or you may need to learn to say 'No' (*see* Step 8 about social skills such as assertiveness).

➤ Taking breaks (whether from chores, family, or a 10-minute break from work) can help. Plan some regular **time-out** to simply relax and enjoy – it is okay to do that, and in fact is really important.

➤ Sometimes taking a **mental break** from a worrying problem is useful – write it down and then put it away. You may even want to allocate 10 minutes of worrying time to it and then say 'that's enough, time to put it away'.

➤ Remember to **nurture** yourself – look after yourself emotionally, and also with good food, rest and relaxation. Are there simple ways that you can reward yourself, for your own reasons (maybe just getting through the week, or achieving one of your goals)? Possibilities are a relaxing bath, a bunch of flowers, seeing a movie or having a massage.

➤ You might like to explore **aromatherapy** – some essential oils, such as lavender, are said to be calming. A couple of drops of the oil can be put in a bath, for example, to gain the benefits of the soothing aroma. Some massage therapists use diluted essential oils in their massage oil – the combination of touch and aromatherapy is very relaxing (see *the safeguards outlined in the section on improving sleep earlier in this step*).

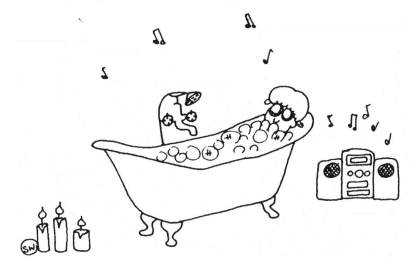

➤ Finding **activities** that you can get involved with, and that occupy and stimulate your mind, can be enjoyable and beneficial (*see* Step 7).

➤ **Humour and laughter** are good stress relievers. So try having a joke with a friend or hire a comedy movie. Sometimes it is a real effort but remember that it can bring about positive effects.

➤ In places like prisons it has been recognised that certain **colours** can have a calming effect on people. Certain shades of pink, blue and violet are reported to be calming. You might like to explore this further. What colours do you find calming? One relaxation technique incorporating colour is available at www.radcliffe-oxford.com/keepingthebluesaway.

➤ Are there any people to whom you can turn for support when you are feeling stressed? Sometimes a good chat and some support is just what is needed. There may be family, friends or acquaintances to talk with, or you may feel you can talk with your GP or MHP, a priest, or community health worker. Write their names and phone numbers here.

Don't forget to ask for help if you are feeling very stressed, and don't feel embarrassed about doing so.

Points to remember
- Stress is part of life. It means different things to different people.
- Stress can be triggered by external or internal factors.
- Stress is a process comprising a stressor, the reaction of the mind and body, and a response.
- The 'fight-or-flight' response is involved.
- Stress can be both a positive and negative experience.
- Stress that persists can cause exhaustion and proneness to illness.
- Identifying situations which cause stress, and factors within yourself to work on, are important steps in managing stress.
- Strategies for coping with stress include problem- and emotion-focused strategies.
- Identifying how you respond and cope with stress, and what main concerns underlie the stress, is important.
- Don't forget general measures for dealing with stress such as keeping healthy, nurturing yourself, taking breaks and doing enjoyable activities.

AVOIDING ALCOHOL, CIGARETTES AND OTHER DRUGS

Some difficulties related to using various drugs have been discussed earlier in this manual. These include:

1. misusing drugs such as alcohol or marijuana, which are risk factors for depression
2. increased smoking and drinking being a risk from depression itself
3. self-care being important; this includes moderating alcohol and cigarettes and not using illicit drugs like marijuana and amphetamines
4. sleep, which is often troubled in depression, not being helped by caffeinated drinks such as coffee, or alcohol
5. stress and anxiety also being worsened by caffeinated drinks and smoking.

It is worth checking your alcohol intake. A standard drink is a drink containing about 10 g of alcohol; for example, this is found in 285 mL of regular beer or 100 mL of wine (note wine is often served in large glasses often containing up to 200 mL).

It is advised that men have no more than four drinks a day, and avoid drinking on two days of the week. For women two drinks a day is the maximum, with two alcohol-free days a week.

If you or your family are concerned about your use of alcohol, cigarettes or other drugs, please speak with your GP. They can provide further assistance or advice on how to access appropriate help.

GAMBLING

Sometimes gambling can become a problem when you are feeling depressed or anxious. Gambling can cause distress, worsened anxiety and depression, and financial difficulties. If you are feeling anxious or depressed about gambling, or your family is concerned, please speak with your GP or MHP. They can support and assist you, and expert help is also available in the community.

Remember, help is available.

NOTES PAGE

Useful coping skills

'I'm still learning' (Michelangelo)

KEEPING A MOOD DIARY

It can be useful to keep a diary of your mood (Greenberger, 1995). You can record what is happening with your mood each day by completing a mood scale; rate your mood on a scale of 0 to 10, where 0 refers to no depression, and 10 to the most severe depression. Use the same diary to comment on:

➤ your sleep length and quality, and what your eating is like

➤ significant events or activities of the day.

The diary will help you be more aware of what is happening and be a good basis for discussion with your GP. The diary for one week will look like this:

	DAY 1	DAY 2	DAY 3	DAY 4	DAY 5	DAY 6	DAY 7
Mood (0–10)							
Sleep							
Eating							
Other e.g. events, changes to medication							

As time passes you will see progress. As things improve, try to focus on positive feelings and events. What helped you pick up in mood, no matter how simple a thing? What positive events have happened in your life, no matter how small? What positive shifts are happening in your life – are you sleeping better, or becoming more active?

PROBLEM SOLVING

When feeling stressed or depressed, negative thoughts can seem overwhelming. It can be harder to think through a problem clearly, and to know where to start in dealing with it. One practical strategy that can help is called 'structured problem solving' (Andrews and Hunt, 1998; Huibers, Beurskens, Bleijenberg, *et al.*, 2003; WHO, 1997). This sounds complicated, but it isn't. Problem solving is a good way to become more self-reliant.

Problem solving **involves sorting out what the problems are and looking at logical, practical ways of dealing with them**. It involves a number of tasks, with the aim of deciding on the best possible solution for the problem. This may not be a total or perfect solution, but it will be a start and it will usually be helpful and make a difference.

Here are the **general rules** for problem solving.

1. When learning the technique of problem solving, start with more straightforward problems rather than complex ones.
2. Set aside time without distraction to help you think clearly.
3. Deal with problems one at a time.
4. Go through each task one at a time.
5. When making a list of possible solutions, write down all your ideas even if some seem wild – in the end you will need to choose an achievable solution, but the process of writing down all the possibilities often generates good ideas.
6. When planning how to carry out the solution, be realistic – are the resources (time, money . . .) available?
7. Include plans on how to deal with difficulties or negative responses that might arise (such as looking at what went right and what went wrong, and what alternative strategies could be used; acknowledge disappointment but plan to try again).
8. Think about how you might manage positive outcomes, as these might involve adjusting to change.
9. As with goal setting, it is useful to set a time by which to carry out the solution.
10. Remember that even partial success is a win, and the process of problem solving is a learning process (WHO, 1997).

(Look back to Step 2 of this guide on goal setting, and have another look at these rules. You can see that some of the principles of goal setting apply to problem solving too.)

The tasks involved in problem solving are
- define the problem in everyday terms
- make a list of all possible solutions
- evaluate the solutions; that is, think about the advantages and disadvantages of each solution
- choose the best possible solution
- plan how to carry it out – this involves breaking the solution down into steps
- review your progress.

On the following page, there is a sheet that you can photocopy and use for problem solving. Your GP or MHP can look at some examples with you.

PROBLEM SOLVING

TASK 1.

Define the problem – that is, write down in your own words what you think the problem is.

_____

_____

_____

_____

TASK 2.

Make a list of all the possible solutions to the problem.

_____

_____

_____

_____

TASK 3.

What are the advantages and disadvantages of each possible solution?

1. _Advantages_   _Disadvantages_

2. _Advantages_   _Disadvantages_

3. _Advantages_   _Disadvantages_

TASK 4.

Based on the solution that seems to have the most advantage rather than disadvantage, choose the best possible solution for now.

_____
_____
_____
_____

TASK 5.

Do some planning – what steps will you need to do to carry out this solution?

1.

2.

3.

4.

5.

(Plan as many steps as you need)

TASK 6.

Review how the problem solving is going. What has worked and been achieved? What still needs to be worked on?

_____
_____
_____
_____
_____
_____

(Adapted from Andrews and Hunt, 1998.)

Getting on with things and not procrastinating

In Step 1 the symptoms of depression were listed. They include loss of motivation and lethargy – it can be very hard to do anything, even get out of bed, when depressed. But there is a link between what you do and how you feel, so it is worth working on not-procrastinating, that is, getting on with things.

In his book *Feeling Good: the new mood therapy*, David Burns talks about a **lethargy cycle**. In this cycle self-defeating thoughts such as 'things are too difficult, there is no point', are linked to self-defeating actions such as avoiding the day and staying in bed. They are also linked to **self-defeating** emotions (helplessness, worthlessness, feeling overwhelmed). Inactivity and low productivity results, along with feelings of inadequacy. Self-confidence suffers.

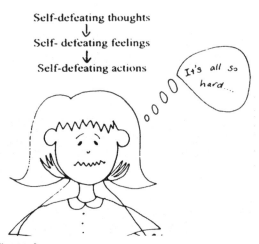

Self-defeating thoughts
↓
Self-defeating feelings
↓
Self-defeating actions

It's all so hard....

(Burns, 1999; Tanner and Ball, 2001)

Sometimes procrastination is related to expecting too much of oneself. **Perfectionists often defeat themselves by setting very high standards.** Many students procrastinate and are late with an assignment because they expect it to be perfect. Procrastination may also result from fear of failure, that is, thinking that putting in an effort and not succeeding would be a terrible defeat. Not everyone succeeds at everything, and not everyone fails at everything.

We know, however, that **activity brightens mood** (Hickie, Scott, Ricci, *et al.*, 2000; Kidman, 2006). So now is the time to get started. In this section a useful strategy called 'daily activity scheduling' will be explained. In Step 7 the benefits of activity in general, and choice of activities, will be looked at in greater detail.

Daily activity scheduling is about **restoring** some **normality** in life. Normal routine and daily activities are often lost in the early stages of depression. Activity scheduling is also about gaining a greater sense of **control** and **satisfaction** in life. It can help you manage your day and make better use of your time.

Here are some **guidelines** for planning your activities.

1. Don't plan for the whole week at once, just take one day at a time.
2. Plan the activities one day ahead.
3. Plan them in one-hour time slots.
4. Try and plan some activities that give you pleasure.
5. Start with easy-to-achieve activities, and gradually include more difficult tasks.
6. Don't worry if you miss an activity. You can still continue with other scheduled activities.
7. Note any extra activities that were done throughout the day.
8. Work towards getting back to a more normal routine, and try the 'activity scheduling' for at least a week (Burns, 1999; Tanner and Ball, 2001; WHO, 1997).

An activity scheduling chart is given on the following page. It can be copied for use.

To **get started** you can try just working on one activity per day. It may be getting out of bed or having a shower, or it may be going for a walk. Build up your level of activity gradually. Encourage yourself with thoughts, such as 'let's give it a go', or 'it might be hard to start with, but it will get easier once I get going'. Once you are doing more, try to include more activities that give you pleasure and a sense of achievement. You might write down meeting a friend for a coffee or going to an exercise class, for example.

The *pleasure and achievement ratings* refer to the degree of pleasure and achievement you associated with the activity. Use a scale of 0 to 5 with 0 for no pleasure/achievement and 5 for very high pleasure/achievement.

Points to remember
- It is useful to keep a diary of your mood.
- As things improve try and focus on positive feelings and events.
- Problem solving is a useful practical strategy. It involves sorting out what the problems are and looking at logical, practical ways of dealing with each of them.
- There can be a lethargy cycle in depression. Self-defeating thoughts, feelings and actions can be linked.
- Perfectionists often defeat themselves by setting very high standards.
- Activity brightens mood. Daily activity scheduling is another practical strategy to restore some normality in life.

Activity Schedule:

DATE _____ TIME _____	PLANNED ACTIVITIES	TICK WHEN DONE, OR NOTE OTHER ACTIVITIES	RATE BOTH PLEASURE AND ACHIEVEMENT (0 TO 5 FOR EACH)
7–8 a.m.			
8–9 a.m.			
9–10 a.m.			
10–11 a.m.			
11–12 p.m.			
12–1 p.m.			
1–2 p.m.			
2–3 p.m.			
3–4 p.m.			
4–5 p.m.			
5–6 p.m.			
6–7 p.m.			
7–8 p.m.			
8–9 p.m.			
9–12 p.m.			

(Burns, 1999; Tanner and Ball, 2001; WHO Collaborating Centre for Mental Health and Substance Abuse, 1997)

RELAXATION TECHNIQUES

In Step 3 on healthy lifestyle one of the issues discussed was stress. Relaxation techniques were mentioned as one of the ways of dealing with stress. **There are physical and mental benefits from relaxing**. These include potentially positive effects on blood pressure and the immune system, improved sleep and reduced anxiety.

Everyone can learn to relax more and gain the benefits. Relaxation is a positive experience in different ways. It tends to be confidence boosting and gives a sense of control. Relaxation techniques are part of a holistic approach to health and are especially important to learn in depression and anxiety. A range of basic techniques will be covered here. Don't expect to be an expert initially. Be patient and try them – you may find one technique suits you better than another.

How long should you allow to relax? You might want to set aside 20 or 30 minutes initially. As you become more familiar with the techniques you tend to relax more readily and less time is needed. Don't let time be an excuse – even five minutes of relaxation is useful.

[Note – *People with a psychotic illness, such as schizophrenia, should not use these techniques as the psychological condition could worsen. If you have strong emotional issues right now, talk with your GP or MHP about them. They can advise you as to whether or not the techniques are appropriate to use.*]

Physical relaxation

One of the first forms of relaxation to learn is physical relaxation. You may or may not be aware of areas of tension in the body already. Some people hold tension in muscles of their foreheads, jaws, or neck and shoulders. Some hold it in their abdomen.

When muscles are tense they tighten and become shorter in length. The body can get used to holding that area in a tense state. When muscles relax they lengthen and become looser and more comfortable.

Simple stretches can help loosen tight areas *[only do stretches that you feel that you can manage physically]*. Sometimes it is good to do a few stretches before you settle down to do the other forms of relaxation.

In Step 3 the 'windmill stretch' was explained. An alternative is to simply reach upwards with your arms and push up onto your toes and stretch to the sky.

Use the following techniques to loosen the head and neck and shoulder areas in particular:

➤ Move your forehead muscles up and down, smile, loosen the jaw.
➤ Gently and slowly move your chin down towards your chest, and hold for a few seconds, and then move the head gently back *[never push further than is comfortable]*.
➤ Move your head gently and slowly to one side (with the ear moving towards the shoulder) and then the other.
➤ Gently roll your shoulders forward a few times and then roll them back.

Progressive muscle relaxation is another way to relax physically (Davies, 2000; Hickie, Scott, Ricci, *et al.*, 2000). This technique is available at www.radcliffe-oxford.com/keepingthebluesaway. Sit or lie in a comfortable position, go to the toilet beforehand, make sure that you are warm enough, loosen any tight clothing, make sure your legs and arms are uncrossed and if wearing glasses, remove them. Let your eyes close. Allow 15 to 20 minutes initially for this form of relaxation alone.

Relax the following areas by being aware of any tension in them and **letting go** of it. Feel the muscles loosen and lengthen.

➤ Relax the muscles of the face (forehead, around the eyes, in the cheeks, around the mouth, in the jaw area).
➤ Relax the scalp and the neck, especially the muscles at the back of the neck.
➤ Loosen across the shoulders and down into the shoulder blades.

➤ Relax the muscles of the upper arms, the forearms, into the hands and fingers.
➤ Let the chest muscles relax.
➤ Relax the muscles of the back, all the way up and down the spine.
➤ Relax the tummy muscles and the buttock muscles.
➤ Let relaxation flow down into the legs, through the thigh muscles, calf muscles and into the feet.
➤ Enjoy the feelings of physical relaxation for as long as you want to, open your eyes when you are ready and return to your day.

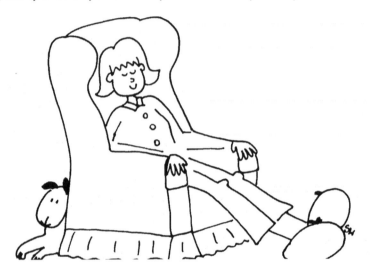

Breathing techniques

Another key in learning to relax is to breathe effectively (Singh, 1996). When stressed, for example, the breathing rate can increase and breathing can become shallow. The usual resting breathing rate in an adult is about 12 breaths per minute, but when anxious it may go up to 25 breaths per minute.

Try this range of breathing techniques and find out what suits you.

➤ Breathe in and out through your nose if comfortable with this, or in through the nose and out through the mouth. Simply be aware of the breath in and then the breath out. Breathe at a gentle slow pace, and feel the cooler air moving in. Breathe out and feel the warmer air. Say 'relax' as you breathe out, and let go of tension and stress as you do so. (This technique is available at www.radcliffe-oxford.com/keepingthebluesaway.)
➤ **Abdominal breathing** or diaphragmatic-type breathing. Effective breathing means expanding your chest by lowering your diaphragm – in doing so the abdomen moves outwards. The larger volumes of the lungs are at the bases of the lungs.
➤ Often we think a 'deep breath in' means raising the shoulders, but this is where the smaller volumes of the lungs are.

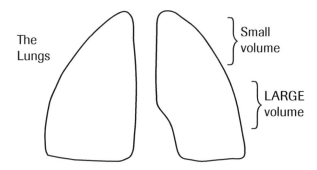

Try abdominal breathing while sitting or standing or lying (depending on what suits you). Place your hands over your abdomen – let them relax. Breathe in and feel the hands rise, breathe out and feel them fall. Repeat. Make an effort to pause and breathe in this way several times during the day.

Practise this technique with your GP or MHP.

Once you feel more confident with each of the progressive muscle relaxation techniques and a breathing technique, you can combine the two. Breathe and relax as you relax each of the areas of the body, or start with one and then do the other.

Visualisation

Are you able to picture things in your imagination? Some people can and other people find this more difficult. If you are able to visualise, then following on from physical relaxation, you may want to try a visualisation technique.

Choose a special and safe place that is peaceful and relaxing to imagine. It may be curled up in a chair with a book, or it might be walking along a beach. Imagine being in that special place and doing what you enjoy. You can have a person or a pet with you if you want, always peaceful and safe. Get in touch with the different sensations such as the feel of the breeze, the smells, or the colour of the sky.

Don't worry about thoughts that may come into the mind – let go of any concern about them and let them drift past.

In this special place it is good to give yourself some encouragement. People often find **affirmations** helpful – these are statements about what you can do or feel or achieve, said in the present tense – such as 'I am feeling more relaxed each day', 'my self-confidence is growing day by day'.

If you are not able to visualise, that is all right. Simply be in the moment and deepen the feeling of peace. Some people listen to music when they relax and focus on the music. Take the opportunity to encourage yourself with affirmations.

In Step 3 the role of colour in relaxation was mentioned. There are some very pleasant relaxation techniques based on colour (Hunter, 1988). A relaxation technique involving colour is available at www.radcliffe-oxford.com/keepingthebluesaway.

Whenever you are ready to finish the relaxation, whatever form you use, gradually head back to the present moment by reorienting yourself to where you are and the day. In the audio track, counting from one to five is used to allow a few moments to reorientate yourself.

Other relaxation ideas

➤ **Meditation** uses techniques to empty the mind of thoughts. When the mind is quiet, the body also relaxes. Meditation techniques are often taught in the community – try contacting your local community health centre or council.

➤ The term **'mindfulness meditation'** is often used. This refers to learning to direct one's attention and energy to where it is needed (Hassed, 1996). It is about being very much in the moment and not struggling with unnecessary mental activity. You can apply mindfulness to meditation or to any simple daily task (Thich Nhat Hanh, 1987).

➤ There are meditations that focus on healing, which can be comforting and helpful. The colour meditation in the audio track incorporates healing.

➤ Different forms of meditation may be used by people with different **spiritual beliefs**. You may have an interest in exploring these, or you might not. Buddhist teaching includes meditation, for example, while Christian teaching focuses on prayer.

➤ **Yoga** is an activity that incorporates body stretching and relaxation. You may find that it suits you. Classes are often held locally, so have a look in the local paper.

➤ **Tai Chi and Qigong**, which originated in China, are moving meditations. They incorporate breathing techniques and are very relaxing. Again the local paper is a good source of groups in your local area.

➤ **Hypnotherapy can be valuable** in learning how to relax and deal with anxiety (McNeilly, 1996). Suggestions can be given to aid confidence and reinforce helpful thinking in depression. Some GPs and MHPs are trained in hypnosis.

➤ **Simply getting out into the garden or walking** (especially at the beach) can be very relaxing. You can use your relaxation techniques at the same time, or simply enjoy nature and explore your senses – the smell of the flowers or sea air, touching a tree or sand at the beach.

Points to remember
- There are physical and mental benefits from relaxing.
- Everyone can learn to relax more and gain the benefits.
- Enjoy physical relaxation, breathing techniques and visualisation.
- Other relaxation ideas include meditation, yoga and tai chi.
- Hypnotherapy can be valuable in learning how to relax.
- Simply enjoying your garden or walking can be relaxing.

DEALING WITH PANIC EPISODES

This section is for those experiencing panic attacks with the depression. A **panic attack** is defined as a **'discrete period of intense fear or discomfort'**, and may include any of the following symptoms.

- palpitations (pounding heart or fast heart rate)
- excessive perspiration, shakes and tremor
- feeling breathless or like you are choking
- chest pain or tightness
- nausea or abdominal symptoms
- dizziness or feeling faint
- feelings out of touch with reality or 'out of your body'
- feeling out of control
- a feeling of impending doom or death
- tingling or numbness (in the hands or feet, or around the mouth)
- hot or cold flushes

(Mental Health Foundation of Australia, 1998)

During a panic attack, the individual will often try to leave the situation hoping that the panic will stop. Others may seek help in case they have a heart attack or go crazy.

Treatment involves the following

➤ Further **education** about panic attacks. Your GP can answer any questions on panic attacks, and there are several useful books listed under 'Resources' in the final step of this guide.

➤ **Reassurance** is important. Remember that **stress is part of life and anxiety is a normal human emotion**.

The physical symptoms are part of the body's normal reaction to danger. But in anxiety the symptoms are out of proportion to the situation, and a panic attack is like a false alarm – there is not actually any danger. Panic is an extreme form of anxiety, which is frightening, but it is **not dangerous**. You feel distressed with panic, but you will not come to any harm. Also, having panic episodes does not mean you are losing control or going crazy.

➤ **Support** from family and friends. There are also community groups, which provide education and support (*see* Resources in Step 10).

➤ Learning **coping strategies** for dealing with panic attacks. These include learning to control many of the physical symptoms through breathing, learning how to deal with situations in which panic attacks have occurred (and that you might be avoiding), and challenging negative thinking associated with panic. More will follow on these strategies.

➤ **Accepting** the situation and knowing that the symptoms will pass. Do not get frustrated or guilty. You will master coping strategies with practice and these will help you prevent panic.

➤ Using the **relaxation techniques** explained earlier in this step.

➤ **Slowing down** – don't rush. Plan the day and do one thing at a time.

➤ **Caring for yourself**. Review healthy lifestyle issues in Step 3. Avoid too much caffeine, and exercise regularly if possible.

➤ Identifying and dealing with any **underlying causes** of anxiety, such as relationship difficulties, is important. You can seek assistance from your GP or a mental health professional in this regard. They can put you in touch with community services that may be able to help.

➤ Thinking about **what has helped in the past** and using these strategies.

➤ **Carrying a card** in your purse/wallet that reminds you about strategies to use when having a panic episode, and perhaps has some reassuring words or a phone number of a support person to call. Here is an example.

Things that help when I feel panicky:
breathe and relax
'I'm okay', 'The feelings will pass'
no unhelpful thoughts
distract myself, e.g. count backwards from 10
have a glass of water, not coffee
call my friend Jane if I need a chat
look after myself today and do some relaxation.

➤ **Medication** at times. Some antidepressant medications help to relieve anxiety and panic, and the decision as to whether medication is needed is up to you and your GP.

(Barlow, Ellard, Hainsworth, *et al.*, 2005; Fox, 1997; Ham, 2005; Mental Health Foundation of Australia, 1998; WHO, 1997)

Specific strategies to cope with panic
Breathing

➤ When we breathe, the oxygen that all cells of the body need is inhaled and carbon dioxide is breathed out. One of the most distressing aspects of the anxiety response in panic is the effect on breathing, known as hyperventilation.

➤ **Hyperventilation** is breathing at a faster rate than is needed. You may experience feeling breathless and find yourself taking short rapid breaths. The breaths are often shallow, but may be gasping breaths. The result is that there is a fall in the level of carbon dioxide, which produces many of the physical symptoms in panic, such as dizziness and tingling. Because the breathing is ineffective there is a slight fall in oxygen that also contributes to the symptoms, such as an increase in heartbeat or feelings of unreality. Overbreathing is hard work and you may feel hot and sweaty and tired. The chest may feel tight and sore because the muscles are working hard.

How do you recognise hyperventilation? Do you:
➤ feel breathless when you have a panic attack?
➤ notice that you sigh or yawn a lot?
➤ ever take big gulps of air?
➤ find yourself taking short rapid breaths?
➤ if so, you are probably experiencing episodes of hyperventilation (Barlow and Craske, 2006)
➤ you can also **time your breathing** Most people breathe at a rate of 10–12 breaths per minute. Is your breathing rate greater than this?

How do you prevent hyperventilation? The following slow breathing exercise can help. You can use it at the first sign of a panic attack, but it is important to practise it regularly so that you feel confident with it.

Slow breathing exercise.
● Stop what you are doing, slow down and relax.
● Breathe in and out slowly (through your nose if possible). Take medium breaths, not deep breaths.
● Breathe in a 6-second cycle. That is, breathe in to the count of 3, and then out for the count of 3 (in your mind you can say 'in, 2, 3 and out, 2, 3'), which will give a breathing rate of around 10 breaths per minute.
● As you breathe out it can also be helpful to say 'relax' in your mind.
● Try to use abdominal breathing (outlined in Step 4).
● Continue until the panic symptoms have settled.

(Hickie, Scott, Ricci, et al., 2000; World Health Organization Collaborating Centre for Mental Health and Substance Abuse, 2000)

Challenging negative and fearful thinking associated with panic
➤ First of all, when panic attacks occur it is easy to **misinterpret the symptoms** as being dangerous or a sign of a serious problem. As discussed, they are part of our reaction to stress or a threat (refer back to the 'fight-or-flight' response in Step 3).
➤ What happens then is that the symptoms of panic become feared. The symptoms themselves trigger anxiety – it is a **'fear of fear'** situation.
➤ Some of the **common fears** associated with panic are fear of having a heart attack or dying. The symptoms are different and panic is not dangerous. You will not die from panic.
➤ Another fear is of 'going crazy'. Many people experience panic – about 30% of people will have a panic attack at some stage in their life. The symptoms are distressing, but you are not losing touch with reality.
➤ Also, you will not lose control – there have not been any cases of people becoming 'out of control' during panic. You will not hurt anyone or behave dangerously.

➤ Sometimes the fear is around collapsing or vomiting. Nausea is a common symptom of anxiety – it does not automatically lead to vomiting. Collapse is rare in panic. Ask yourself, 'What would be so terrible about vomiting, or collapsing?' We are all human and occasionally these things happen in life – someone would probably be pleased to assist you. They would not be embarrassed and you do not need to be embarrassed.

(Mental Health Foundation of Australia, 1998; World Health Organization Collaborating Centre for Mental Health and Substance Abuse, 2000.)

Let's now look at the role these fears, along with negative thinking, play in worsening panic.

➤ With your GP or MHP, work through what your initial symptoms of panic are, what thoughts occur and the associated feelings.

➤ It may be helpful to keep a diary of panic episodes – when they occurred, what you were doing, your thoughts and feelings. Or you may prefer to work from memory.

Here is an example.

SYMPTOM	THOUGHTS	FEELINGS
Heart palpitations	Oh no, here it comes	Afraid
Short of breath	It's getting worse	Anxious
Light-headed	What if I pass out – and no-one helps me?	Panicky

This is called a **cascade effect**. You can see how a symptom triggers a thought, the thought triggers fearful feelings and the panic worsens. There are some common fears, but we are all individuals and our thoughts and feelings will differ. Now talk through and document a panic episode, and identify *your* particular symptoms, thoughts and feelings.

SYMPTOMS	THOUGHTS	FEELINGS

Looking at a panic attack in this way helps establish **how to tackle your individual panic episodes.** Consider the role of:

a. understanding the symptoms and avoiding misinterpretation

b. challenging the thoughts that lead to more fear. Replace a catastrophic thought like 'I'm having a heart attack', with something like 'I understand the symptoms, and I'm okay – I can cope'

c. slow breathing techniques
d. relaxation techniques
e. visualisation – of a peaceful place, or floating calmly past the panic
f. distraction – for example, the breathing technique is distracting, counting is distracting, as are positive thoughts or visualisation.

(Aisbett, 1993; Fox, 1996; WHO, 1997)

(Note – the book, *Living With It: a survivor's guide to panic attacks*, by Bev Aisbett, is highly recommended. It illustrates these coping strategies very well, in a light-hearted but useful way.)

Learning how to deal with situations in which panic attacks have occurred

➤ One of the consequences of having a panic episode in a particular situation is that you may then try to **avoid** that situation in future.
➤ This is how **phobias** develop, such as agoraphobia, which is a fear of being unable to escape if a panic attack occurs (Sadock and Sadock, 2007).
➤ The way to deal with this is to gradually expose yourself to these situations again in a step-by-step way. This is the basis of a behavioural strategy called **graded exposure**.
➤ With your GP or MHP work out a list of situations that are stressful, or that you avoid as a result of the panic.
➤ Then select some factors that would decrease or increase your fear. For example, going in a lift might be more stressful when travelling many floors, with lots of people or when you are in a hurry. It may be less stressful when travelling a few floors, with a friend or when you are not rushed.
➤ Generate a list of possible situations, and then rank them from least difficult to most difficult. This will give you a series of steps to follow. A brief example follows.

SITUATION	DIFFICULTY (0–10)	STEPS
• Travelling in a lift, several floors, alone	7	1. Lift, one floor only, with a friend
• Travelling in a lift, one floor only, with a friend	4	2. Lift, one floor only, alone
		3. Lift, several floors, alone
• Travelling in a lift, many floors, many people	10	4. Lift, many floors, many people

➤ Your GP will help you devise a program, but yours will involve more steps than in the example above. It is best to progress in small achievable steps.
➤ Plan to tackle the least difficult situation first. Anxiety will initially rise when facing this situation, but it will then fall. Practise this step until it causes little anxiety (at least 50% improved) and then move onto the next.

SITUATION	DIFFICULTY (RANK 0–10)	STEPS

Remember that you have a number of tools to help you tackle each situation – slow breathing, relaxation techniques and challenging your thinking. (World Health Organization Collaborating Centre for Mental Health and Substance Abuse, 2000).

Points to remember
- A panic attack is a discrete episode of intense fear or discomfort.
- Treatment involves education, explanation and reassurance that panic is not dangerous.
- Coping strategies include breathing, learning how to deal with situations in which panic occurs, and challenging negative thinking.
- Use relaxation techniques, don't rush, and take care of yourself.
- Deal with underlying causes of anxiety, and use what has helped in the past.

NOTES PAGE

Helpful thinking or cognitive strategies

'There is nothing good or bad, but thinking makes it so' (Shakespeare)

INTRODUCTION TO COGNITIVE-BEHAVIOURAL THERAPY

In Step 2 **Cognitive-behavioural Therapy** (CBT) was introduced as an effective means of tackling symptoms of anxiety and depression. CBT involves changes in our behaviour and thinking. It is a very practical therapy, is useful in everyday life, and deals with current problems and ways of coping. Most people find that it makes a lot of sense.

Some CBT strategies have already been looked at. Examples of *behavioural* strategies are graded exposure (used in dealing with fears) and relaxation training (*see* Step 4), while an example of a *cognitive* strategy is problem solving (also outlined in Step 4).

CBT takes time and effort. Allow time for the strategies to help and for your thinking to gradually change. As a result your mood will improve. Keep working at the strategies and going through the exercises.

In this step the focus will be on strategies that are helpful in dealing with thinking changes that occur in depression. The thinking is negative, and is often **self-blaming** and self-critical. There can be a **negative view of the world and the future** (Blackburn and Davidson, 1995).

The concept that **the way we think affects how we feel** was introduced in Step 2. Learning how thinking and feeling interact, and how to develop different ways of thinking, is the basis of the cognitive part of CBT. The relationship between thinking, feeling and behaviour is shown below.

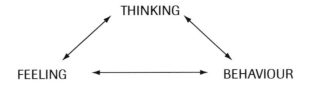

What you *think* affects how you feel and how you *feel* affects what you think. What you *do* impacts on how you feel and think. Going out for a walk in the sunshine, for example, may lift mood.

The following table highlights some of the interactions between thinking and feeling and behaviour.

	SITUATION	FEELING	THOUGHT (OR SELF-TALK)	BEHAVIOUR
Positive interaction	Waking up	Happy	What a nice sunny day	Go out in the sunshine for a walk
Negative interaction	Waking up	Depressed	Another day – things are bound to go wrong – why do I bother?	Withdraw into self, stay in bed

Our minds are busy most of the time. We have a lot of thoughts that occur automatically, and the way we respond to everyday situations is often based on habit. **Automatic thoughts** may be positive such as 'I'll give it a go', or negative such as 'I'll never be able to do it' (Tanner and Ball, 2001). Automatic thoughts are not necessarily a problem, but they may be unhelpful and interfere with handling everyday activities.

Sometimes it is easier to identify feelings before thoughts. Use the list below to help you do this.

POSITIVE FEELINGS	NEGATIVE FEELINGS
Loved	Sad
Happy	Insecure
Joyful	Vulnerable
Amused	Guilty
Excited	Scared
Content	Panicky
Cheerful	Anxious

STEPS TO TACKLE UNHELPFUL THINKING
** There are five steps to tackle the unhelpful thinking that can occur in depression**
(Based on Beck, 1990; Burns, 1999; Davies, 2000; Greenberger and Padesky, 1995; Tanner and Ball, 2001.)
1. keeping a thought diary
2. understanding thinking errors
3. identifying thinking errors
4. challenging unhelpful thinking
5. developing more helpful thoughts.

1. Keeping a thought diary

The first step is to notice in your everyday life how thinking and feeling interact. Become more aware of the automatic thoughts that occur when you are feeling depressed or feeling well. It can be useful to record them. You may have kept the *mood* diary as part of Step 4, when scoring from 0–10 was used (0 meaning no depression and 10 meaning the most severe depression). *Thinking* now needs to be recorded. This is a *thought* diary, and it might look like this:

DAY 1	SITUATION	WHAT YOU WERE FEELING? (NAME FEELING AND RATE ON A SCALE OF 0–10)	WHAT YOU WERE THINKING?	WHAT DID YOU DO?
WORST MOOD				
BEST MOOD				
DAY 2				
WORST MOOD				
BEST MOOD				

Talk with your GP or MHP about how your thinking and behaviour (what you were doing) interacted with your mood. Talk about your worst mood and your best mood. It may help to think about particular incidents that were associated with feeling depressed or feeling good, and keep this diary for several weeks (you could write it in your journal).

2. Understanding thinking errors

The next step is to understand that we all have unhelpful thinking at times – every one of us. In CBT we talk about irrational or illogical thinking. Irrational thinking distorts reality and causes many problems. Some of the common thinking distortions or errors are listed in the following table.

THINKING ERRORS	DEFINITION
All-or-nothing ('black-and-white') thinking	There is no middle ground. Things are seen in black and white; for example, if you make a small error at work, you see yourself as a failure.
Overgeneralisation	Because something has gone wrong in the past, you see a continuing pattern of defeats – 'I always mess things up'.
Jumping to conclusions	You make a negative interpretation of things; for example, you may interpret that someone is thinking negatively about you when there is no evidence of this – 'they think I'm a loser' (mind reading); or you may presume that things will turn out badly (fortune-telling).
Catastrophising	This is overemphasising the importance of events; a small mistake may be perceived as a disaster.
Mental filter	This means dwelling on one single negative thing, to the exclusion of all else.
Disqualifying the positives	Discounting any positive experiences and maintaining a negative outlook.
Emotional reasoning	You feel bad, so this is seen as reflecting how things really are.
'Should' statements	This is about motivating yourself with 'shoulds' and 'musts'. It is about setting high expectations for yourself, and the emotional results may be guilt, frustration or anger.
Labelling	This is giving yourself a label and follows on from overgeneralisation; for example, making a mistake results in thinking 'I'm a loser'.
Personalisation	You assume responsibility for a negative event that you did not cause – 'it's all my fault'.

(Burns, 1999; Tanner and Ball, 2001)

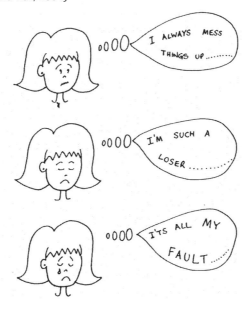

(**Note** – David Burns' book *Feeling Good: the new mood therapy* has a good chapter on thinking distortions, as does *Beating the Blues* by Susan Tanner and Jillian Ball.)

3. Identifying thinking errors

Now you can begin to identify thinking errors. Let's add another column to the thought diary to help you do this.

DAY / SITUATION	WHAT YOU WERE FEELING? (0–10)	WHAT YOU WERE THINKING? (AUTOMATIC THOUGHTS)	THINKING ERRORS

4. Challenging unhelpful thinking

The fourth step is to learn to challenge unhelpful thinking.

   Here are some ideas on how to do this.

   a. Recognise that **thoughts are not facts**; they are actually assumptions.

b. **Look for evidence** to prove or disprove your thinking; for example, get feed-back from other people or consider past experience.
c. **Put the situation into perspective**. Try the following ideas.
   * Look for other explanations – 'Is there another way to think about this? For example, 'It's not fair', may be challenged with 'Unfair things happen to everyone, not just to me'.
   * Imagine talking with a friend with the same issue – how would you advise them?
   * Test out the thinking by gathering information and asking others.
d. **Change the words** used in the thought.
   * For example, 'I should have done better' can be reworded or reframed as 'I did the best I could on the day – I'll keep working on things and next time do better'.
   * Avoid using labels, for example 'I'm a failure' or 'I'm hopeless'.
   * Use flexible words such as 'I would like to' rather than 'should' or 'must'.
e. **List the advantages and disadvantages** of the thought. Is the thought helpful or unhelpful? Does it work for you or against you?

5. Developing more helpful thoughts

Now work on developing more realistic and helpful thoughts. The table below gives examples of common thinking errors in depression and anxiety, and some more helpful ways of thinking.

COMMON THINKING ERRORS IN DEPRESSION:	MORE HELPFUL WAYS OF THINKING
All-or-nothing, or black-and-white thinking: for example, 'I'll *never* be able to manage', or 'I *have* to get *top* marks'.	Change your perspective by considering other possibilities, such as 'I may have some trouble managing, but I can cope', or 'I don't have to be perfect'.
Overgeneralisation: for example, 'I always mess things up', 'I never get it right'.	Look for evidence to disprove your thinking – think about the times you *did* 'get it right', or ask other people what they think. What are the facts?
Labelling: 'I'm hopeless.'	Avoid naming yourself. Use different words such as 'There are things I did well today, and I will work on the things that I want to do better'.
Catastrophising: 'It's a disaster', 'What if I never meet anyone else?'	Work on a more balanced outlook – there is no reason to think the worst is likely to happen. Ask yourself what the most likely outcome is going to be. Questions like 'Is it the end of the world?' or 'Am I exaggerating?' can be helpful. Avoid 'what ifs' – consider that something may be possible, but not actually probable.

(*continued*)

COMMON THINKING ERRORS IN DEPRESSION:	MORE HELPFUL WAYS OF THINKING
Disqualifying the positives: for example, 'They implied that I could have done better'.	Check whether you are discounting positive things that were said. Ask yourself, 'Am I only considering the negatives?'
Personalisation: for example, 'It must be my fault'.	Ask 'Am I blaming myself for things that are not my fault?' Avoid inflexible words such as 'must'.

(Burns, 1999; Tanner and Ball, 2001)

It may be useful to make a card to carry around with you with examples of helpful statements or the sorts of questions you can ask yourself to challenge any negative thinking.

Helpful thoughts and questions

For example:

    is this thinking helpful?

    what evidence is there?

    is this 'all-or-nothing' thinking?

Use the table below to work on developing more helpful thinking:

DAY / SITUATION	WHAT YOU WERE FEELING? (0–10)	WHAT WERE YOU THINKING? (AUTOMATIC THOUGHTS)	THINKING ERRORS

MORE HELPFUL THOUGHTS	WHAT DID YOU DO?	OUTCOME (FEELING 0–10)

Points to remember

- CBT is a useful and effective way to tackle symptoms of anxiety and depression.
- The way we think affects how we feel.
- Automatic thoughts may be positive or negative.
- Follow the five steps to tackle the unhelpful thinking that can occur in depression:
  - keeping a thought diary
  - understanding thinking errors
  - identifying thinking errors
  - challenging unhelpful thinking
  - developing more helpful thoughts.

A COUPLE OF IMPORTANT ISSUES IN CBT FOR DEPRESSION
Where do thinking errors come from?

As we go through life we develop **assumptions and beliefs** about the world, others, and ourselves. Beliefs operate at an unconscious level, but come into play when we need to respond to situations. Just as you have learned to identify automatic thoughts, you can learn to identify underlying beliefs.

The psychological theory is that we can develop a number of **unhelpful or irrational beliefs** (Blackburn and Davidson, 1995). In depression, beliefs tend to be negative. They may relate to needing to be loved by everyone or needing to be 100% successful – otherwise 'I'm a failure'. In anxiety the beliefs relate to a sense of being threatened and lacking the ability to deal with threats; for example, 'I should always watch out if I am to avoid something awful happening' or 'If I feel anxious, this means I am losing control'.

The following table lists a number of unhelpful beliefs and gives alternative, more helpful views.

UNHELPFUL BELIEFS	MORE HELPFUL VIEW
All significant people in my life must love me and approve of me.	I would prefer to be liked by people but there is no way I can guarantee it.
I must always be competent, adequate and achieving in every area of my life.	No one can be like that all the time – I accept my strengths and weaknesses.
My life should progress easily and smoothly. Things should work out the way that I want them to. It's awful when things go wrong.	Things are not necessarily going to go as I want. I will do my best to overcome obstacles, but if that isn't possible I will accept their existence.
My life experiences determine how I feel. How can I feel good when things don't go as they should?	Depending on how you view the world, individuals can be sad or disappointed.

(*continued*)

UNHELPFUL BELIEFS	MORE HELPFUL VIEW
It is better not to take risks, because when you stick your neck out, you can get easily hurt.	If you don't take sensible risks you will never know whether something is enjoyable or not. See uncertainty as a challenge.
I must always be in control of situations.	The world is full of chance, but life can be enjoyed despite this. Wanting perfect control leads to a sense of loss of control.
People should be sensitive to my needs and do what I believe is right.	People's sensitivity varies greatly, and they are generally looking after their own interests. I can be assertive about my needs.
The world should be a fair place. I must always be treated fairly.	I would prefer it were fair, but there is injustice in the world. I will do my best to encourage fairness but accept that it often won't be fair.

(Kidman, 2006)

Just as you have learned to develop more helpful thinking, you can work on your beliefs too. **Awareness** is the first step.

In their CBT program *Mind Over Mood*, Dennis Greenberger and Christine Padesky make the following suggestions to help identify underlying beliefs.

Identify **themes** from your thought diaries. Can you identify themes that may suggest underlying beliefs about yourself, others or the world? An example might be being a failure or not lovable. Are you a perfectionist, expecting a lot from yourself?

A **'downward arrow technique'** – taking a situation and a thought and then asking yourself 'What does this say or mean about me?' Repeat this question until you get to the heart of the issue. For example:

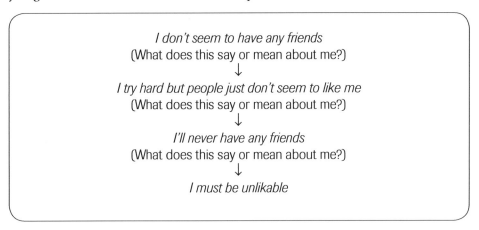

Depending on the thought it may be more appropriate to ask 'What does this say or mean about others . . . or about the world?' With your GP or MHP look back at the tables in this step and look at this technique to identify unhelpful beliefs.

Once you have identified an unhelpful belief, make a list of its **advantages and disadvantages**. You may well find the disadvantages outweigh the advantages. Another way of thinking about this is to weigh up how the belief works *for* you and how it works *against* you.

You can then challenge the unhelpful thinking relating to these beliefs.

For example, how does procrastinating, caused by believing that you must always do a fantastic job, work *for* you? How does it work *against* you? Procrastinating may mean that you do a very good job, but become extremely stressed in the process.

As suggested by Bev Aisbett in her book *Living With It*, be a friend to yourself. This might mean giving encouragement to yourself. One way of doing this is through **affirmations.** These are positive statements about how one can think or feel or behave. Examples are: 'I am feeling calmer and more confident each day' or 'I don't have to be perfect – we are all human.'

Consider a couple of affirmations that best apply to you and think of them each day, maybe during relaxation. Write down the affirmations you have chosen.

_____

_____

_____

_____

_____

Dealing with being a perfectionist

You have probably met someone who is a perfectionist, or maybe you are one yourself. Being a perfectionist means wanting to do things extremely well. People who want to do a good job are often quite productive – the trouble is that perfection is not possible, and putting pressure on yourself to do everything perfectly causes stress and defeat.

In his book *Feeling Good: the new mood therapy*, David Burns speaks of perfection as being an illusion. He writes that it does not exist in the universe – everything can be improved, and striving for perfection causes disappointment.

Have a look back at the list of unhelpful beliefs – which ones do you think might drive perfectionism?

_____

_____

_____

Being a perfectionist is often about wanting approval – perhaps it is thought that others expect a perfect job and high achievement. Perfectionists may define their self-worth by how well they perform. Sometimes it is about wanting to feel in control – but the reality is that things cannot be totally controlled.

How to be less of a perfectionist (Burns, 1999; Tanner and Ball, 2001)

1. Be aware of expectations – your own and others. Question whether they are realistic.

2. Doing things perfectly does not make people value you or approve of you more. It can, however, wear you out!

3. Weigh up the advantages and disadvantages of being a perfectionist. You may want to keep some of the advantages, and let go of some of the disadvantages, or you may find that there are more disadvantages and decide to change how you do things.

4. Try lowering your standards a little, for example, aim to do a *good* job instead of a *perfect* job. You may be surprised at the effect. Frustration and procrastination are likely to decrease, and you may well find that satisfaction increases. You will even create some time to relax.

5. Establish some limits on what you do – for example, in terms of time you might spend on a task.

6. Be aware of fear that might hide behind perfectionism – maybe fear of failure or criticism. Fear can maintain unhelpful behaviours, and the way to deal with fear is to challenge it. You may want to do this one step at a time (*see* Step 4) and get some support from a friend or your GP to help you.

7. Recognise that you *can* change – avoid saying, 'I can never change' or 'I always have to do the job this way'.

8. Keep things in perspective.

9. Work out some questions to challenge your thinking around being perfect. These might be examples.
   - 'Who says that I must always be perfect?'
   - 'What would happen if I made a mistake occasionally?'
   - 'Would it be the end of the world?'
   - 'What is the worst that could happen?'
   - 'Would that be so terrible? Could I live with that?'

10. Remember, very few things are perfect. It is okay to be average. In fact, challenge yourself to be mediocre!

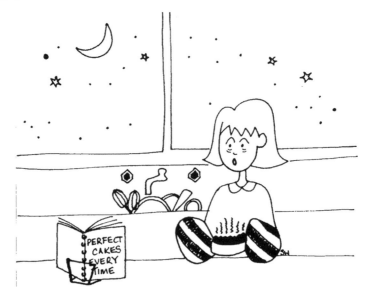

MINDFULNESS-BASED CBT

It is known that negative thinking styles contribute to depression relapse. When feeling sad, automatic negative thinking styles can be triggered (Segal, Williams and Teasdale, 2002). A vicious cycle occurs in which sad feelings and negative thoughts reinforce each other (*see* Step 1). Therefore, it is vital to tackle negative thinking early if there are signs of relapse (Segal, Williams and Teasdale, 2002).

To do this, one needs to be mindful of one's feelings and thoughts. **Mindfulness** refers to paying attention to what you are doing and experiencing the present moment (Segal, Williams and Teasdale, 2002). Mindfulness means paying purposeful attention, not being judgemental and being in the here and now (Kabat-Zinn, 1990). For example, if you are washing the dishes or reading a book, mindfulness means being totally aware of and involved in the moment.

The mindfulness principle can be readily applied to thinking. Psychologist Joseph Hinora speaks of observing thoughts just as if you are standing at a bus stop watching different buses come and go. Each bus represents a different thought and you can observe them (even see the thought written on the front of the bus). You have choices about getting onto a bus or not. In the same way, you may choose to go with the thought or let it go.

This sort of technique is part of mindfulness-based cognitive-behavioural therapy (MBCT), which combines cognitive and meditation techniques. MBCT can have a number of positive consequences.

1. Awareness enables a person with depression to realise when they are about to undergo a downward mood swing.
2. Being aware weakens the depressed thought.
3. It enables the person to halt the vicious cycle between negative thoughts and feelings (Segal, Williams and Teasdale, 2002).
4. It is a gentle approach that also pays attention to feelings and budding sensations (such as tension).

A brief mindfulness-based meditation is available at www.radcliffe-oxford.com/keepingthebluesaway. You are guided to be aware of the body and your breathing, to focus on simply being, and to observe your thoughts. Once aware of thoughts linked with depression-relapse, you can challenge them, let them go, or you might choose to do a pleasant activity to help lift your mood (*see* Step 7).

A positive aspect of MBCT is raising awareness of pleasant events and feelings that occur during the day. MBCT can help you achieve a sense of balance in life.

It is worthwhile practising mindfulness in your everyday life. Take a few moments during the day to be truly mindful – are your neck and shoulders tight and can you relax them? Really listen to people; enjoy the sunshine or a pleasant view.

ACCEPTANCE AND COMMITMENT THERAPY

Acceptance and commitment therapy (ACT) is a recent behavioural therapy, which places a major emphasis on the development of mindfulness skills. It aims to help the individual handle painful thoughts and feelings, and to create a rich and meaningful life. Rather than evaluating thoughts, it encourages us to view thoughts as a series of words or stories (Harris, 2007).

ACT is based on a number of core elements, namely:

➤ defusing unhelpful thoughts (for example, singing them!)
➤ expansion – making room for unpleasant feelings
➤ connection – living in the present (being mindful)
➤ observing your thoughts (for example, 'I am having a thought that . . .')
➤ clarifying and connecting with your values
➤ committed action; that is, creating a rich and meaningful life through effective action (Harris, 2007).

KBA touches on some of these elements over the 10 steps of the program. It is suggested that further reading about ACT, or working through the core elements of ACT with a GP or MHP, be undertaken to follow on from the KBA program. *The Happiness Trap: stop struggling, start living*, by Dr Russ Harris, is recommended.

NOTES PAGE

Dealing with psychological issues

'What lies behind us and what lies before us are tiny matters compared to what lies within us' (Ralph Waldo Emerson)

Individuals will have their own personal and psychological issues to work through. This step addresses a number of psychological issues that may be experienced by individuals with depression. There may be other issues that you will decide to discuss with your GP, MHP or support person.

SELF-ESTEEM AND DEPRESSION

Self-esteem refers to how you see and judge yourself, often in comparison to others. It describes one's sense of self-worth. In CBT terms it relates to our underlying attitudes and beliefs about ourselves. Self-esteem includes, but is more than, *self-confidence* (beliefs about our ability). Your sense of self-worth affects how you function generally and how you relate to other people. *Self-acceptance* is another important aspect of self-esteem.

Many individuals with depression express low self-confidence or self-dislike, even self-loathing. The founder of CBT, Dr Aaron Beck, found that 80% of people with depression expressed self-dislike. He spoke of feeling 'defeated, defective, deserted and deprived' in depression (Beck, 2008).

In *And Light at Last: recovery from depression* on Internet Mental Health (1998), the author 'Louise' describes the huge impact of depression on self-esteem. Sufferers 'cease to like or to love themselves', and come to believe they are worthless, hopeless and helpless. This is one of the most damaging aspects of the depression. In managing depression, it is very important to work on the issue of self-esteem (Dryden and Mytton, 1999).

Early life experiences can affect self-esteem. A child who is constantly criticised by others, for example, is not going to develop a strong sense of self-worth. Our self-esteem is affected by the society in which we live, and we are all in some way influenced by the media, culture, government, and education. The influences may be positive or negative.

Unhelpful thinking, as discussed in Step 5, is a major influence on self-esteem. All-or-nothing thinking is a real trap. It can lead to labelling yourself as a failure, for example, which can be self-defeating. Why try new things if you see yourself as likely to fail? (Burns, 1999)

Tanner and Ball (2001) write about 'beliefs that rob people of self-esteem'. These include the following.

- I must keep proving myself through my achievements.
- I must do things perfectly.
- I must have everyone's approval.
- I need to be loved to be worthwhile.
- The world must be fair and just.

They go on to talk about challenging these beliefs.

➤ **Our worth is not actually about what we achieve**. Achievements give a sense of satisfaction, but not true self-esteem. Focusing on achievement means focusing on the future rather than now.

➤ Perfectionism and the disappointment it can lead to was explored in Step 5.

➤ We all seek approval from others. You have to be careful not to measure your sense of worth based on the expectations or the praise of others. **What is really important is what you think about yourself,** whether you accept yourself and what you do.

➤ We all feel a deep need to be loved. Burns (1999) writes that most people are in fact loved by others, but what is missing is **self-love.** We have to watch that we don't base our sense of self-worth on being in a relationship.

➤ Unfortunately there is suffering in the world and things are not always fair. We don't always get what we would like, and need to be **realistic and flexible**. Work on **patience and acceptance.**

Do you have any other ideas about beliefs that might interfere with self-esteem? Write them down.

_____
_____
_____
_____
_____
_____
_____

Ways to improve self–esteem

➤ Reflect on how your early experiences in life have affected your self-esteem. How does society influence how you view yourself?

➤ Use CBT (*see* Step 5):
1. identify unhelpful automatic self-critical thoughts
2. challenge them
3. replace them with more positive responses.

It is always useful to write them down initially – use three columns, as shown below. Remember to remove the 'shoulds', 'musts' and 'if only' statements.

SELF-CRITICAL THOUGHT	THINKING ERROR	MORE HELPFUL THOUGHT
I never do anything right	Overgeneralisation	Actually, I do a lot of things right
It shows what an idiot I am	Labelling	I'm not an idiot

A technique that has proved useful over many years in clinical practice comes from a book by Hillman (1992) called *Recovery of Your Self-Esteem*. This technique involves three steps.
1. **Recognise your positive points and strengths** by making a list of 'What I like about myself: my positive points'. Reflect on this list and add to it over time; maybe ask others for ideas. Read the list regularly and acknowledge your positive points. Contemplate them when you meditate.
2. **Recognise the 'inner critic'** or the inner negative voice and make a list of 'Things I do not like about myself: negative points'. Consider whose voice is being critical – has the criticism been internalised from other people?
3. Then **reassess** these negative things and be fairer on yourself. Are the statements too critical? Can they be re-worded so they are less harsh? Try reframing the statements into goals – an example would be 'I tend to be quiet in front of others, but I am working on talking with people more'.

Remember that our positives and negatives can be like two sides of a coin. A strength, such as being determined, can also be a negative at times – determination might be interpreted as stubbornness. Reinforce your strengths with positive self-talk such as 'This is a strength' and 'I can manage this'.

Here are three tables to use for this exercise:

What I like about myself: my positive points

Things I don't like: negative points

Rewrite the negatives

➤ Think about children; it is clear that each one is special and unique. Children grow up into adults, so remember that **each individual is special**

and unique. Consider your uniqueness. What things about you make you unique? It doesn't matter how small or mundane these things seem at first glance. It might be that you have freckles or a special smile. You might enjoy collecting stamps or reading thrillers. Maybe there is something special or unique about your personality. Jot ideas down in your journal, or use the space below to record your ideas.

> **I am a special and unique person!**

Celebrate your successes and achievements, *and* your uniqueness.

➤ The book *How to Stop Worrying and be Happy* (Gressor, 1996) speaks of **letting go** of the things that you don't like about yourself. It suggests that you:
  - *look outward* to see that others make mistakes too
  - *look inward* and learn from any mistakes
  - *look forward* because you cannot change what has happened, but you can decide how to live in the present and learn for the future.

All good advice!

➤ Other tips are:
  - know and use your abilities
  - set realistic goals for yourself
  - develop your strengths. You will find that confidence in one area tends to spread into other areas
  - don't compare yourself with others (remember that everyone has their own strengths and weaknesses)
  - ask for help with things if you need to. That's okay. And have patience with yourself. Everything takes time
  - learn to enjoy your own company and sense of independence
  - develop your own interests.

(Burns, 1992; Kidman, 2006)

➤ A colleague once said that when she feels low and lacking self-esteem, she focuses on what it is like to be feeling better and more confident. This gets her back to feeling more positive. Sometimes she pretends that she is feeling confident, and this helps lift her too.

➤ **Self-respect** is important. Try treating yourself as you do others, and don't put yourself down. Be compassionate to yourself. Nurture yourself and be a friend to yourself. This can mean allowing yourself to enjoy some pleasurable activities – jot down a list of possibilities in your journal, and revisit goal setting (Step 1) to make some plans for pleasure. Pleasurable activities can be a great reward for effort. Nurturing yourself also means looking after your health and well-being (*see* Step 3).

➤ **Develop creativity**. Doing something creative is a great way to boost self-esteem. It is very rewarding to create something, whether it is a special meal, a poem or artwork (*see* Step 7).

➤ Finally, but most importantly is **self-love.** This is the aim – accepting and loving yourself for who you are. Burns (1999) explains in *Feeling Good: the new mood therapy* that at 'the bottom line, only your own sense of self-worth determines how you feel'. The need for approval is strong in some people – not everyone is going to give us approval, but we can give ourselves self-approval. Eleanor Roosevelt was very wise when she said, 'No one can make you feel inferior but yourself'. We may learn to be self-critical but this can be unlearned.

➤ There is an excellent book by Choquette (2008), about loving yourself and living consistently with your spirit which encourages the reader to be aware of what their passions are, and to honour themselves and their passions.

➤ McMillen and McMillen (1996) wrote a book called *When I Loved Myself Enough*, which is a series of contemplations about loving one's self. One of the very important messages they give is that **when you love yourself, you come to realise that you are special and unique, and life becomes simpler.**

Points to remember

- Self-esteem refers to how you see and judge yourself.
- One of the most important tasks in dealing with depression is raising self-esteem.
- Early life experiences can affect self-esteem.
- Our worth is not based solely on what we achieve.
- What is really important is what you think about yourself.
- We need to be realistic and flexible, and practise patience and acceptance in life.
- To improve self-esteem:
  - reflect on the influence of early experiences and society
  - use CBT techniques
  - recognise your positives and reassess your negatives
  - remember that each individual is special and unique
  - let go of the things you don't like about yourself, and learn from mistakes
  - develop your strengths
  - self-respect is important
  - develop creativity
  - aim for self-acceptance and love.

LOSS AND GRIEF AND DEPRESSION

The information presented in this section on loss and grief is largely based on the work of grief expert, Dr Sheila Clark, and the Graduate Program in Grief and Palliative Care Counselling at the University of Adelaide in South Australia.

As mentioned in Step 1, **depression may be triggered by loss in life**. Loss may be **death-related or non-death-related** (Bowlby, 1980). We may grieve the death of a person or pet. An example of a non-death-related loss would be divorce, or loss of one's job or health. 'Attachment' between individuals develops to maintain a state of balance in life (Bowlby, 1980). Loss and grief disturbs this balance – people often describe a sense of their 'whole world being thrown upside down'.

Grief is the response to loss, and affects many aspects of the individual – **physical, emotional, behavioural, cognitive** (such as memory and concentration), **social and spiritual.** It involves adaptation to the loss, and as loss threatens our inner assumptions about the world, it takes time to re-adjust (Corr, 1998; Parkes, 1988).

Loss may be hidden by individuals, particularly if there is stigma or shame involved. Loss may be gradual, such as adapting to dementia in a parent. There may be differences between men and women in grieving, or cultural differences. Individuals may not seek help with their grief because of these factors.

Sometimes individuals can become stuck in their grief and an intense grief reaction continues (Rando, 1984). This can be related to unresolved feelings such as guilt. An ongoing or long-term grief is called **chronic grief** (Middleton, Burnett, Raphael, *et al.*, 1996; Parkes, 1998).

Grief is accompanied by sad and low feelings. **Many of the symptoms experienced in normal grief overlap with symptoms of depression,** such as sadness, crying, loss of appetite, disturbed sleep and poor concentration. However, these symptoms gradually lessen over time. On some occasions though, a depressive illness may develop. This is when depressive symptoms are both prolonged (more than two months) and more severe than expected (American Psychiatric Association, 2000; Davies, 2000).

Depression itself may cause losses, such as loss of health, social contacts or ability to work. These losses in turn may add feelings of grief to the depression. Depression can be a hidden illness, due to the stigma associated with mental health problems. What losses have resulted from your depression?

_____

_____

_____

_____

Grief work

Adjusting to loss **takes time** and effort. It can be very useful to talk with your GP or MHP or a friend. It is important to find someone who is a good listener and someone whom you trust. There has been a lot written about grief work, and there are a number of different approaches to grief therapy. Several approaches providing a holistic way of dealing with loss and grief will be highlighted here.

Grief therapy approach of Worden (1982, 2008, as cited in Payne, *et al.*, 1999).

➤ **Understanding** the process of grief, and that it is normal to have positive as well as negative feelings about the lost person or object.

➤ **Sharing** thoughts and feelings about the loss and reviewing what it means to the individual. It can be helpful to look at photographs or mementos of the lost person together, for example.

➤ Identifying and **expressing** negative emotions associated with the loss – such as self-blame or anger. One way to do this is to talk about things that we miss or don't miss about the person.

➤ **Problem-solving** ways of coping with the troublesome feelings resulting from the loss, practical problems, or new ways of coping in life (*see* Step 4).

➤ Eventually **letting go** of attachment – this does not mean giving up on the lost person or object, but rather 'finding an appropriate place' for them in our emotional lives.

Dr Sheila Clark's advice.

1. Allocating **grief time** each day – say 15 to 20 minutes in which to have a cry or write about the loss (such as in your journal).
2. **Naming the problems** – emotional or practical.
3. Looking after general health – endeavouring to eat regularly, and avoiding overindulgence in alcohol or smoking.
4. Taking time out to walk in the park.
5. Sometimes spoiling yourself, for example, having a coffee with a friend, or relaxing in a hot bath.
6. Not making any major decisions before at least one year has passed.
7. Continuing existing relationships, seeking support.
8. Getting some advice on dealing with practical issues, or dealing with special occasions such as Christmas or the anniversary of the loss.
9. Understanding that your ability to think and remember is reduced – don't be too hard on yourself, and use reminder lists.
10. Considering whether you need some time off work or to negotiate reduced working hours.
11. If possible, finding some meaning out of the loss, such as growing in strength as a result (Clark, 1995).

There are also a number of strategies for dealing with **negative thinking** that can occur in grief. Fear, guilt, anger, sadness, self-blame or blaming others can all occur in grief. The principles of CBT outlined in Step 5 can also be applied in the context of loss and grief.

➤ Be aware of your thinking (keep a thought diary).

➤ Identify thinking errors, for example, all-or-nothing thinking ('I'm hopeless – I can't manage everything.') or catastrophising ('What if I lose someone else?').

➤ Challenge unhelpful thinking.

➤ Work on developing more helpful thoughts.

Sometimes **thoughts can be intrusive** in grief. You may not want to deal with them at the time (it may not be an appropriate time to have a cry, for example), or just need a break from them. Try imagining putting the thought aside, perhaps into a box on a shelf. You can then come back to it later, such as in your grief time, and deal with it.

Note too that **self-esteem can be adversely affected** through loss and grief. Be aware of this and work on raising your self-esteem.

Reviewing progress can be a powerful tool in recovering from a loss – could you have coped as well three or six months ago, for example? What resources have you found within yourself that have helped you cope?

A number of factors which help individuals adjust to loss have been identified (Gamino, Sewell and Easterling, 2000). At some stage, **achieving a sense of closure** is important. This generally refers to closure with the physical body after a death, but it does not include closure to the love and influences of the person who died. Letting go of the lost person or object can be difficult, and tends to happen gradually – part of this may be gradually giving away the deceased person's belongings. Sometimes there are still things that need to be said to the deceased, and it can help to say these at the graveside or in a poem or letter.

Narrative therapy speaks of 'saying hullo again' to the deceased, rather than saying goodbye (White and Denborough, 1998). This refers to incorporating what has been lost into the present, for example, holding on to the influence (or some other aspect) of that person that is meaningful. Although someone may no longer be alive this does not mean they no longer exert influence. What would they have said or done in certain situations? Can you see their characteristics in your sibling or child for example?

The other factors include **creating positive memories** of the lost person or object. (Note – if the person was abusive this may not always be appropriate.) You may choose to look at photos and talk about the loss. Creating a special scrapbook or memory box with photos and mementos can also help. Focusing on what was special about the person and the things they brought into your life is part of discovering **meaning**.

Consider **what you have learned** through the loss – have you grown in any way, developed strengths or discovered true friends? What about **spiritual beliefs**? There are studies that indicate that spiritual beliefs assist in resolving grief (Walsh, King, Jones, *et al.*, 2002). Spirituality can be based on differing beliefs, but usually 'it places one's relationship with a higher power at centre stage and uses a religious creed to organise life events and experiences' (Allport and Ross, 1967). Have your beliefs been challenged, changed or strengthened?

You may want to write down your thoughts about what you have learned, how you have grown, or how your spiritual beliefs have helped or been changed.

_____

_____

_____

_____

_____

_____

Consider looking at relevant websites such as Grieflink (www.grieflink.org.au), undertaking reading or courses on relationship loss, or asking well-known funeral directors about grief work in groups. There are many good books available on grief.

Points to remember
- Adjusting to loss and grief takes time.
- It is important to understand the process of grief, and share thoughts and feelings about the loss.
- Allow 'grief time' each day.
- Look after yourself.
- Take time out.
- If possible find some meaning out of the loss.
- Challenge unhelpful thinking related to the grief.
- Self-esteem can be affected in grief.
- Achieving a sense of closure is important.

THE 'NEGATIVE' EMOTIONS AND DEPRESSION

We all experience a range of emotions, including **anger, guilt, shame, jealousy and hate.** These are often referred to as 'negative' emotions. This does not mean they are 'bad', but they can have an adverse affect on how you feel about yourself or others. Emotions such as anger may be expressed in unhelpful ways, such as through aggressive behaviour or withdrawal. These behaviours can lead to more difficulties, and so the aim is to learn to express these emotions in helpful or constructive ways.

The first step in dealing with any of these emotions is acknowledging that they exist. This involves learning to recognise and name the emotion (Burns, 1992; Greenberger and Padesky, 1995).

About anger and jealousy

Anger is what you feel when provoked. The emotion of anger ranges from irritation to rage. It is accompanied by physical reactions such as tight muscles and increased heart rate – remember the 'fight-or-flight' response explained in Step 3? Well, this is the fight part! The anger reaction is also accompanied by thoughts and behaviours. Anger does not have to lead to aggression. It can have a positive function, such as energising you to express yourself (Greenberger and Padesky, 1995).

In terms of thinking and anger, look back to Step 5, especially the part about beliefs. Anger can be linked to thinking that we have been treated unfairly (this will vary between people), or prevented from obtaining something we expected to achieve. In relationships, anger is often related to unfulfilled expectations of the other person. It is important to consider how realistic those expectations are, and whether they have been clearly communicated to the other person.

Anger is a normal response to many situations. It is a normal part of grief, for example. There are close associations between anger and depression, and you may find that you move between the two. If an individual has been abused in the past, they may be alert to more abuse and become angry when feeling threatened. Chronic anger may be experienced (Greenberger and Padesky, 1995).

You need to consider whether the anger is a problem for you.

➤ Do you get very angry?
➤ Do you stay very angry?
➤ Do you act aggressively?
➤ Does anger interfere with your work or relationships? (Montgomery and Morris, 1989)

If so, learning skills for managing anger will be very important for you.

In *Beating the Blues* (2001), Tanner and Ball describe two types of jealousy – the envious type ('I wish I had . . .') and the possessive type, which stems from fear of loss. Possessive jealousy can impact negatively on relationships, whether with a friend or partner. There may be underlying insecurity or low self-esteem.

Managing anger

➤ Can you identify the **underlying reasons** for the anger? Sometimes we are angry for different reasons than we think. It might help to ask yourself, 'What do I really need or want?' (And if there is conflict with someone else, what do they really need or want?) Do you need reassurance, or are you tired and stressed and need some help? (Scott, 1990)
➤ **Accept responsibility** for the part of the anger that you own. External factors play a significant part, but how we interpret them and how we control the anger are also very important.
➤ Identify and recognise your own **early warning signs** of anger, for example, muscle tension or black-and-white thinking. Know what coping strategies work for you, and put them into place.
➤ Monitor your level of anger, and use self-talk. When you feel anger building up, tell yourself to take some **time out** or remove yourself from the situation. This allows you to get back in control of your emotions and prevent the situation from escalating (Scott, 1990).
➤ Put the anger aside and **deal with the problems**. See the problem-solving technique outlined in Step 4.
➤ Use the anger as a sort of drive to take positive action to bring about change.
➤ **Anticipate** events that are likely to trigger anger and prepare yourself. What will you say? How will you remain calm and in control? Rehearse

the situation in your mind and give yourself encouragement about coping (Greenberger and Padesky, 1995).

➤ Work on **understanding the thinking associated with the anger**. Stop and record the situation, your mood and thinking. Or recall a situation in which you felt angry and identify the thoughts that you had.

➤ Review what you learned in Step 5, and challenge the unrealistic or unhelpful thinking. Anger is often triggered by catastrophising the situation, black-and-white thinking, believing the situation is unjust, or blaming yourself or others. Replace thinking 'it's not fair and it's their fault' with 'bad things happen at times', or 'they couldn't help it' (Tavris, 1989).

➤ Beware of always needing to be right or in control of others. This may stem from insecurity.

➤ Try helpful self talk, such as these examples.
  • 'Yes, I am angry. I'll notice what I'm thinking.'
  • 'I can handle the situation calmly.'
  • 'Breathe and relax, then deal with the situation.'

➤ You can apply the same cognitive principles to dealing with **conflict in relationships**.
  • Be aware of thinking errors that can worsen conflict, such as black-and-white thinking ('you always . . .') or mind-reading ('you think . . .').
  • Avoid generalising in arguments – stick with the central issue rather than also including other things you think are a problem.
  • Avoid resurrecting old issues over and over; avoid labelling yourself or the other person ('I'm . . .'or 'You're . . . useless'); and avoid blaming ('It's all your fault').

➤ **Communicate effectively** if the anger is related to others. Listen to the other person and encourage them to listen to you. You both need to be able to express yourselves and understand the other's position. Consider what you need to say and how you can express it clearly. Look at the person and speak firmly. Say what upset you about what the person did (be specific), and tell the person how you feel. Then suggest how the situation might be prevented from happening in the future.

➤ Note that **being assertive is different to being aggressive**. Learning assertiveness skills can be really helpful (explained in Step 9).

➤ A useful strategy, developed by Adelaide psychologist Lindy Petersen to assist with parenting, can be applied to dealing with anger. It involves traffic lights! We are all familiar with red for stop, orange for caution and green for go.
  • Remember to stop (red) and think. What is the problem and how do you feel? What is going on for you and for the other person?
  • Take your time and be cautious (orange) before you act. What could you do? What are the options and what might happen with each of these?
  • Once you have made your choice and decided what to do – whether that is taking time out or expressing your anger – then go ahead (green) and act constructively (Petersen, 1992).

➤ **Look for the positives** in people and situations (Montgomery and Morris, 1989).

➤ Is it possible to **let go** of some or all of the anger, and find compassion in yourself to forgive the other person or the situation? It may seem a very big ask of you, but it may help you feel better in yourself (more about this later).

➤ Work on **accepting** that sometimes other people do not have the capacity to change or act differently. Accepting this may help you move on.

➤ **Rest and relaxation** can help. Sometimes you get a new perspective on the situation after a rest or sleep. Try the relaxation techniques outlined in Step 4. Breathing and relaxing can be particularly helpful.

➤ **Let off steam** through exercise, talking with a friend, or expressing yourself creatively. Throwing and shaping pottery clay, or even play dough, can be very therapeutic. So can punching your pillow.

➤ Can **humour** help – is there a funny side to relieve some of the tension? Or perhaps taking some time out and finding something to laugh about might help (for example, watching a comedy).

➤ Finally, when **dealing with another person's anger** it can help to communicate effectively, by listening and speaking clearly. Empathy statements can help the other person tell you about their anger – an example is 'I can see you're very angry. Can you tell me about it and help me to understand why?' Suggest time out if the anger is escalating, and make sure that you feel safe.

Managing jealousy

➤ Sometimes jealousy is triggered by low **self-esteem** and feeling insecure as a result. Work on building your self-esteem (*see* earlier section on self-esteem in this step).

➤ Avoid comparing yourself to others. Remember we are all unique individuals.

➤ We all need to be independent, even if in a relationship. Develop your independence and your ability to manage challenges and difficulties using your own resources.

➤ Be aware of the jealous thoughts and challenge them – are they realistic and are your expectations realistic? Replace these thoughts with alternative and more positive **trusting** thoughts.

➤ Remind yourself of more positive experiences (Tanner and Ball, 2001).

Guilt and shame

Guilt occurs when we have not lived up to our own standards, when we think that we 'should' have done things differently. **Shame** is the sense that we have done something wrong, and tends to involve a very negative view of ourselves (Greenberger and Padesky, 1995). Sometimes guilt and shame are quite appropriate, if we have actually done something wrong.

But in depression, the emotions of guilt and shame can be out of proportion to the situation, or quite misplaced. They can be associated with thoughts about being 'bad' or 'worthless'.

Take these steps to deal with guilt and shame.

1. Assess the seriousness of the situation by asking:
   - are you justified in feeling guilty, or is your thinking distorted? (*See* thinking errors in Step 5.)
   - what is the evidence?
   - how important is it in the bigger picture of life?

   You might ask a friend what they think about it.
2. Work out how much responsibility *you* need to take and how much others own – be realistic here, because you may have blamed yourself when you were not actually responsible (for example, we may blame ourselves for things that others did to us as children, when the adult person was really the responsible one).
3. Talk about the situation and the uncomfortable feelings with your GP or a friend.
4. Accept that you are human and that everyone makes mistakes – watch out for unrealistic 'shoulds' and any perfectionistic tendencies, and work on forgiving yourself.
5. Make amends for the part you are responsible for.

(Burns, 1999; Greenberger and Padesky, 1991)

Again, relaxation can help you deal with uncomfortable feelings like guilt or shame – breathe in, and relax as you breathe out. Let go of the 'shoulds'. You are okay!

'LETTING GO' IN DEPRESSION

The potential value of letting go of negative emotions was mentioned earlier. Negative emotions can hold back your progress. You may feel 'stuck' in anger or guilt, maybe from the past, and the emotion may be continuing to get you down.

There is a book by Bev Aisbett (1996) called *Letting it Go: attaining awareness out of adversity*. It is a useful little book, and in part looks at learning to love and forgive others and ourselves. It explains that this takes courage and it helps reduce your own suffering. It can free you up to move on.

Writing in your journal or doing other creative activities may be a good way to gradually express and let go of troublesome emotions.

Another way of enabling you to let go of emotion is via a 'ritual' or ceremony (Bass, 2008). You would be aware of various rituals in our society such as marriages and funerals. These help us prepare for, acknowledge, and cope with changes in life, and sometimes to bring closure to events.

In the same way very simple psychological rituals can help us to let go of emotion which may have been holding us back. They focus on letting go of the negatives, making a time for change and a new beginning (Saunders, 1992).

[Only consider a ritual if you are feeling ready emotionally. Discuss your thoughts with your GP or MHP.]

Here are some *guidelines* for planning your ritual.
➤ Think about the theme of the ritual, and decide your goal.
➤ Take time to plan the ritual carefully.
➤ Keep it simple.
➤ Incorporate elements or symbols in it that are meaningful to you.
➤ Are there things that you particularly want to say or express?
➤ Do you want to have music?
➤ Choose the right time and place – do you want the ritual indoors or outdoors?
➤ How do you want to feel at the end of the ritual? What do you want to be different?
➤ Always end the ritual with something positive.
➤ Take time to reflect afterwards.

Here is an example of a ritual.
A young woman, improving after having had some mental health problems, wants to let go of the remaining guilt and grief. She also wants to celebrate her improvement and what she has learned about herself. She decides to buy some helium-filled balloons, and plans for each one to represent something different. One will represent guilt and another grief. She chooses the brightest coloured balloons to represent her hard work in recovery, and the positive things about herself – her strength and courage. The young woman makes a cake and has a special celebration. She lets go of the balloons representing guilt and grief. The brightly coloured balloons representing positive things become the centre-piece at her table.

LONELINESS AND DEPRESSION

We are social creatures, and relationships are important. In depression there is a tendency to withdraw from people, and feeling lonely can be an issue. You may live alone and feel lonely, or be in a relationship and feel lonely.

Sometimes loneliness and loss go together (Holmes and Holmes, 1993). One may feel lonely because of loss through death or divorce. This is an issue of dealing with loss and grief – the principles outlined earlier in this step may be helpful.

With respect to loneliness resulting from being disconnected from people, it can be useful to check your thinking. For example, you might think that 'no one cares'. But maybe people who have actually been helpful in the past are unaware of the current problems. Are you communicating about the problems? Have they got a lot of their own concerns right now?

Sometimes we compare ourselves to others, and imagine other people lead fabulous lives all the time. For example, a pop star reported enjoying the adulation of an audience and then feeling very lonely when returning to an empty hotel room after each concert. Things are not always how they seem. **Focus on your life and enriching it rather than comparing yourself to others.**

If loneliness is a problem, **do some goal setting** (*see* Step 2). You may decide to work on becoming more active and involved with others. Activity is a great way to lift mood (*see* Step 7) and to meet people, or you may want to work on existing relationships.

HOPELESSNESS, SUICIDAL THOUGHTS AND DEPRESSION

Depression may be associated with feeling hopeless and with thoughts of suicide. There is greater risk of suicide in someone who:

➤ is feeling severely depressed and feeling hopeless
➤ has made plans for suicide, or
➤ who has a family history or past history of suicide attempts (Mann, 2002).

It is very important to talk with someone if you are troubled by suicidal thoughts – a family member, friend, your GP or MHP. Suicidal thoughts can be very frightening and distressing, and just talking about your thoughts can be a relief.

Your GP will assess your level of risk of suicide and work out the best treatment (Horgan, 2002). Sometimes, understanding that others have experienced the same sense of hopelessness and have recovered, helps (Mann, 2002). Sometimes support and treatment by your GP or MHP is helpful, and sometimes advice from a psychiatrist or hospitalisation is needed.

It is important to identify your thoughts and feelings. Is there underlying anger or guilt? Are there thoughts about punishing yourself? Remember things are not hopeless – *there are always solutions to problems*. There are other options to suicide and there are reasons for living (Burns, 1999). You are not alone – **help is available**.

If you are feeling suicidal, keeping close contact with your GP is vital. It is useful to keep a note of what to look out for in your feelings and thoughts, and who to contact in case you feel suicidal (Morgan, Jones, and Owen, 1993). See the Resources section at the end of this guide, or your local phone book for Mental Health Emergency phone numbers.

Points to remember

- We all experience a range of emotions – anger, guilt, shame, jealousy and hate.
- Anger is what you feel when provoked, and can be a normal response to many situations.
- If the anger is a problem, learning anger-management skills can be important.
- Work on understanding and dealing with the thinking associated with the anger, jealousy, guilt or shame.
- Work out how much responsibility *you* need to take and how much others are responsible for.
- Good communication with others is important.
- Letting go of negative emotions can be very valuable.
- Focus on enriching your life and connecting with other people.
- If you are feeling suicidal, talk with your GP. Remember that you are not alone, there are solutions to problems, and help is available.

FINDING HOPE AND MEANING

'Inside myself is a place where I live alone and that's where you renew your spring that never dries up' (Pearl Buck)

The importance of hope

Near the start of this guide it was stated that depression treatments are effective and that 'you will improve'. You were asked to remember that there is light at the end of the tunnel! This was done because of the importance of hope in recovering from depression.

It is important to recognise that the symptoms and problems that you have been experiencing are part of the depression. As the depression improves, many of these resolve. This healing, along with the skills that you are learning and the lifestyle changes that you are making, will help in recovering from depression and staying well in the future.

Unfortunately life does have difficult times and times of suffering. Accepting this, and the ways in which you respond to these challenges are important (Yapko, 1991). That is why you have been asked to work hard on your thinking and emotional responses. It will be important to keep developing your coping skills, positive lifestyle choices, and thinking.

Finding meaning and purpose

People have probably always asked the question 'What is the meaning in life?' There is a counselling approach called existential therapy that is concerned with understanding the person and what it means to them to be alive. This approach considers the person to be in a constant process of learning and change (Dryden, 2002).

Victor Frankl (1905–97), one of the founders of existential therapy, was Jewish and experienced Hitler's concentration camps first-hand. He described three sources of meaning that allowed victims to survive: a life purpose, a love, or a sense of meaning through suffering (Christie-Seely, 1995). He wrote that the essence of being human could be found in the search for meaning and purpose (Corey, 2008).

Existentialism recognises the importance of the physical aspects of oneself, as well as the social, psychological and spiritual (Dryden, 2002). For some people the spiritual aspect may relate to a relationship with a God or higher power; for others it is about finding meaning through nature or within oneself. You may have a particular religious belief, or you may not. Sometimes exploring different religious ideas can be helpful. Spiritual approaches can sometimes help us cope and find meaning, even when facing suffering (Aldridge, 2000).

Buddhism acknowledges suffering in the world, but is optimistic. It recognises the importance of placing less emphasis on ourselves, and more on kindness and compassion. Buddhism advocates that people have a capacity to grow, and meditation is seen as central to this growth (Lafitte, 2002). Christians believe in God and an after-life. For many people these beliefs are central to their lives. Love and compassion are advocated.

The Dalai Lama is sometimes quoted as saying that 'the purpose of our life is happiness'. This is explained further in his book, *The Art of Happiness* (1998). Our task in life is to discard the things that lead to suffering, and accumulate the things that lead to happiness. This is done by gradually increasing our awareness of what truly leads to happiness.

ACT is viewed as having elements of existentialism. It aims to help us create a meaningful life, while accepting the pain that goes with it. It focuses on the individual's values and connecting with a sense of purpose in life (Harris, 2007).

Narrative therapy was referred to earlier in this step and in Step 1. Two approaches used in narrative therapy may be helpful in dealing with suffering and finding meaning. One is externalising the problem – talking about how 'the depression' affects you – recognising that you are not the depression. The other is looking for alternative experiences. Even during very difficult times, people find strength to cope (White, 1998).

Philosophy also provides some helpful observations on happiness. The philosopher Epicurus divided human needs into different categories. The 'natural and necessary' needs include those essential to a safe and happy life, such as food and shelter, clothing, freedom and friends. A meal at an expensive restaurant would be considered 'natural but unnecessary'. Needs that were self-centred, such as fame or power, were considered 'unnecessary'. Epicurus was born in 341 BC, yet these thoughts are just as relevant today.

When considering your own personal fulfilment and happiness, remember to look at all areas of your life – the physical, social, emotional and spiritual (Fenton-Smith, 2002). When you review your goals (from Step 2) from time to time, look at establishing goals in all these areas.

Also, over time, focus on your passions in life and the areas in which you find purpose.

Being thankful

Psychologist Joseph Hinora also advocates thankfulness, or recognising the things that you can be thankful for. These may include things that someone has done for you, or the things that you have received (no matter how small). It may simply mean being thankful for the food that you are eating today, or being thankful for your health, family members or friends.

There is evidence that keeping a weekly gratitude journal (or list of things you are thankful for) can enhance an individual's feelings of happiness (Lyubomirsky 2007). Consider keeping a gratitude journal each week, and writing down what you are grateful for in life, even if it is just someone making you a cup of coffee, or the sunshine (Lyubomirsky, 2007; Reynolds, 2002).

Can you list five things that you are thankful for today?

_____

_____

_____

_____

_____

Inspirational writings

Inspirational quotes have been included at the beginning of most steps in this manual (and sometimes in between). These have been included to stimulate thought and hopefully provide encouragement and inspiration. It is worthwhile looking out for quotes, poems or pieces of writing that have meaning to you as an individual. Sometimes they can help inspire hope, remind us of what is important, or lift the mood and spirits. Here is a poem by Nancye Sims that says some of the important things mentioned in this guide. (Included with permission from the author.)

A Creed to Live By

Don't undermine your worth by comparing yourself with others.
It is because we are different that each of us is special.
Don't set your goals by what other people deem important.
Only you know what is best for you.
Don't take for granted the things closest to your heart.
Cling to them as you would your life, for without them, life is meaningless.
Don't let life slip through your fingers.
By living your life one day at a time, you live all the days of your life.
Don't give up when you still have something to give.
Don't be afraid to admit that you are less than perfect.
It is this fragile thread that binds us to each other.
The quickest way to receive love is to give love;
We deserve to love and be loved.
Don't dismiss your dreams.
To be without dreams is to be without hope; to be without hope is to be without purpose.
Don't run through life so fast that you forget not only where you've been but also where you are going.
Make each day count, life is precious and short.
Life is not a race, but a journey to be savoured each step of the way.

Points to remember
- Hope is vital.
- There are different ways to think about and explore meaning and purpose in life.
- Recognise the things that you can be thankful for.
- Inspirational writing can be very encouraging.

NOTES PAGE

The benefits of activity

'The heavens rejoice in motion' (John Donne)

THE BENEFITS AND JOYS OF ACTIVITY

Activity or occupation is central to life. Our daily routine, our work and leisure time involve activities. Activity provides us with routine, rhythm and balance in life, and can give us a great sense of satisfaction and achievement (Barris and Kielhofner, 1988). Activities also provide us with a lot of fun and enjoyment.

Lethargy and loss of motivation are common in depression. This means the individual with depression is less likely to do the activities that usually provide them with pleasure. A vicious cycle can result – the less active the individual becomes, the more depressed they feel and the less they do (Hickie, Scott, Ricci, *et al.*, 2000; Kidman, 2006).

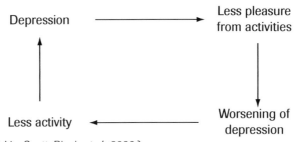

(Adapted from Hickie, Scott, Ricci, *et al.*, 2000.)

Activity is a very broad term that includes a wide range of pursuits – from very physical sports through to gentle activities such as reading and meditation. It is important not only to recognise the importance and benefits of activity, but to **give yourself permission** to enjoy relaxing and pampering activities.

Different people enjoy different sorts of activities. Some people like movement and enjoy things such as sport, walking the dog, scuba-diving or yoga. Some people enjoy auditory activities such as music, and others enjoy visual things such as art. Some activities stimulate a range of senses; think about gardening or cooking – you can enjoy wonderful colours and smells.

Don't forget creative activities, such as art and crafts, as they can be very satisfying. Everyone has creative potential – it is a matter of finding the sort of activity that brings out your creativity. This may be in drawing, music, crafts or writing. Creative activities also allow you to express yourself and build self-esteem.

Some activities are very social – joining a walking group or book club, or taking dancing lessons. You can get to know people in your community by joining a local group or club.

Some activities have great physical health benefits, or incorporate wonderful relaxation such as yoga or tai chi. Caring for a pet can be a great source of enjoyment and occupation. Is there something you would like to learn more about? There are many places to do courses, such as your local community health or adult education centre. Learning can be fun and very satisfying.

People's lives can be greatly changed and their mood lifted through activity. The key is finding activities that are meaningful to the person – perhaps something creative, or doing something to help another person, or teaching a skill.

In his book *The Noonday Demon: an anatomy of depression*, Andrew Solomon (2001) tells a story that demonstrates the power of activity. He writes about a Cambodian woman called Phaly Nuon, who helped many women during the time of the Khmer Rouge. Phaly found many women were depressed and traumatised as a result of the war, and she developed her own way of helping them. She found that helping the women 'forget' the traumas (by hearing the women's stories about other things and using craft and music as a distraction) was helpful. She would then involve the women in activity or work – teaching them skills that they could use in later employment. Finally, Phaly taught the women how to love – beginning with taking care of themselves and each other and in doing so learning how to make friends.

A LIST OF ENJOYABLE ACTIVITIES

Below is a list of of activities. They range from walking to seeing friends, to playing cards or going to markets.

Consider which ones you might enjoy and place a tick next to them. Also add to the bottom of the list any activities not listed that you might enjoy.

Walking
- in your local area
- in the countryside
- at the beach
- with a friend
- with your dog

Riding a bike

Playing sport

Going to the gym

Gardening

Writing letters

Going out for a coffee

Catching up with mates

Going to the library

Searching the internet

Playing computer games

Rearranging a room

Going to a play

Watching a DVD or the television

Listening to the radio

Eating

Cooking

Sewing

Taking a bath or shower

Having a massage

Having a haircut

Talking on the phone

Buying flowers

Fishing

Doing a course

Doing the spring cleaning

Yoga

Tai Chi

Hugs

Going to the cricket

Tinkering in the shed

Reading

Having a cup of tea

Going to the movies

Enjoying a funny film or a good joke

Smiling or laughing

Playing with your children or a friend's children

Seeing friends

Sitting in the sun, or at the beach

Doing crosswords

Swimming

Painting a picture

Making a mosaic

Playing pool

Getting to know your neighbourhood

Going to markets

Sightseeing in your town

Visiting a museum, zoo or art gallery

Going on a day trip

Travelling

Shopping for presents or new clothes

Singing

Playing a musical instrument

Joining a club

Doing a jigsaw puzzle

Playing cards

(Hickie, Scott, Ricci, *et al.*, 2000; Kidman, 2006; World Health Organization Collaborating Centre for Research and Training for Mental Health, 2000)

YOUR IDEAS!

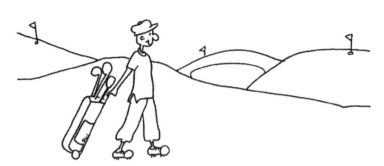

INCLUDE PLEASURABLE ACTIVITIES IN YOUR DAY

In Step 4 we looked at daily activity scheduling, which aims to help restore routine and normality in life. Activity scheduling is also about gaining a greater sense of control and satisfaction in life. It can help you manage your day and make better use of your time. Now that you have thought about pleasant activities, think about ways to incorporate these into your life.

Let's review the guidelines for planning daily activities (Tanner and Ball, 2001; WHO, 1997).

➤ Don't plan for the whole week at once, just plan for a single day at a time.
➤ Plan the activities a day ahead.
➤ Plan them in one-hour time slots.
➤ Try and schedule some activities that give you pleasure.
➤ Start with easy-to-achieve activities, and gradually include more difficult tasks.
➤ Don't worry if you miss or don't complete an activity. You can still continue with other scheduled activities.
➤ Note any extra activities that were done during the day.
➤ Work towards getting back to a more normal routine.
➤ Try the 'activity scheduling' for at least a week.

To get started you can try just working on one activity per day – it may be getting out of bed or having a shower, or it may be having a walk. Build up your level of activity gradually. Encourage yourself with thoughts, such as 'it will get easier once I start'. Once you are doing more, try to include more activities that give you pleasure and a sense of achievement, for example, meeting a friend for a coffee or going to an exercise class.

An activity scheduling chart is given on the following page. It can be copied for use.

➤ The *pleasure rating* refers to the degree of pleasure you associated with doing the activity. Use a scale of 0 to 5, with 0 for no pleasure and 5 for maximum pleasure.

➤ The *achievement rating* refers to the sense of achievement you gained from doing the activity. Again rate it from 0 to 5, with 0 for no achievement and 5 for maximum achievement.

Activity Schedule:

DATE: _____ TIME: _____	PLANNED ACTIVITIES	TICK WHEN DONE, OR NOTE OTHER ACTIVITIES	RATE PLEASURE AND SENSE OF ACHIEVEMENT (0–5 FOR EACH)
7–8 a.m.			
8–9 a.m.			
9–10 a.m.			
10–11 a.m.			
11–12 p.m.			
12–1 p.m.			
1–2 p.m.			
2–3 p.m.			
3–4 p.m.			
4–5 p.m.			
5–6 p.m.			
6–7 p.m.			
7–8 p.m.			
8–9 p.m.			
9–12 p.m.			

(Burns, 1999; Tanner and Ball, 2001)

KEEPING LIFE SIMPLE

'Very little is needed to make a happy life' (Marcus Aurelius)

Focusing on the simple things in life seems to be a good philosophy to live by. Some of the best things in life, like the beauty of nature or a child's smile, are often overlooked.

It pays to keep this philosophy in mind in our very materialistic world. Sometimes we strive for more in life or search for the thing that will provide happiness, when we would be better looking at what we already have. Dr Mark Cohen (2001) writes, 'many people in today's society endure the present, waiting for the promise of future happiness, thinking, "I'll be happy when . . . "' It is important to focus on the here and now.

A patient once said, 'when I started enjoying the simple things again, I knew I was getting over the depression'. The ritual of making a good cup of tea or picking some flowers from the garden can provide a lot of pleasure. Fill your life with little pleasures, focus on the moment and enjoy those pleasures.

LAUGHTER AND HUMOUR

'Laughter is a most healthful exertion' (Christoph Wilhelm Hufeland)

In depression it can be difficult to smile, let alone laugh. However, as the depression improves it becomes easier. There are many reasons to develop the ability to smile and laugh again.

We know that laughter and humour are good for your health. This was acknowledged in the Bible, 'A merry heart makes a cheerful countenance, but low spirits sap a man's strength' (Proverbs 17:22). Eastern medicine has recognised the health benefits for a long time (Cohen, 2001). Laughter is relaxing; it helps the immune system and can help relieve pain (Holden, 1993; Moran, 2002).

Laughter and humour also feel good! And that is reason enough to laugh. Sometimes though, we need to give ourselves permission to feel good. Robert Holden, a British psychologist who began the 'Happiness Project', advocates that we are entitled to feel happy. He actively promotes the benefits of laughter and humour, and suggests:

➤ getting in touch with the ability to play, like a child
➤ using humour and laughter to relieve stress at work
➤ sharing laughter with others
➤ making time for humour and laughter with friends and family
➤ joining a laughter club
➤ smiling more.

Watching a comedy or reading a funny story or a joke book can all make you smile and laugh. *[Warning – some people with asthma find that their asthma is triggered by exuberant laughing. Care is needed.]*

If you have the chance to see it, a BBC production about the Happiness Project called 'How to be happy' is an excellent documentary and has been seen by millions of people around the world. It takes a very holistic approach to improving mood and helping people find more happiness in their lives. The Happiness Project also has a website at www.happiness.co.uk.

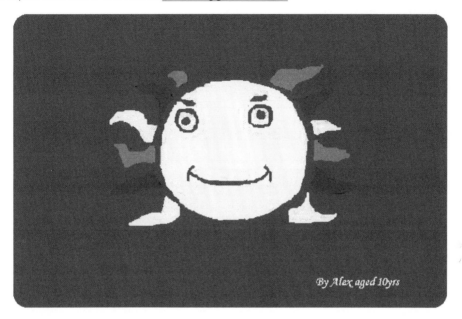

By Alex aged 10yrs

In what other ways can you bring more humour and laughter into your life?

_____

_____

_____

_____

_____

THE ACTIVITY OF GIVING

Once the depression has improved, think about ways to give to yourself and others. There are many different ways to give – even smiling at someone or sharing a laugh is giving. Simple acts of kindness, whether picking up someone's dropped parcel or giving a gift at a time of sadness, can have a large impact.

Giving is a really important part of life, whether it is to family or friends, or to people that you choose to help through volunteering or community service.

Giving is very rewarding. Thinking about others also helps us focus outside ourselves and on the bigger picture in life. The Dalai Lama speaks of kindness and compassion as being important human qualities to develop. He says that his basic belief is that you first need to realise the usefulness of compassion, 'then our life becomes meaningful and more peaceful – happier'.

Points to remember
- Activity is central to life.
- Depression can be helped by activity.
- Give yourself permission to enjoy different activities.
- Include pleasurable activities in your day.
- Keep life simple.
- Smile and laugh more.
- Develop compassion.
- Giving is rewarding.

NOTES PAGE

Fostering social support and skills

'Good company in a journey makes the way seem shorter' (Izaak Walton)

ABOUT CONNECTEDNESS

Step 1 discussed the risk factors for depression and the factors that protect against depression. Having social support (or people around who are supportive) was said to be a protective factor, and having poor social support was said to be a risk factor.

It is generally agreed that social connections play an important role in maintaining a sense of well-being (Kawachi and Berkman, 2001; Spijker, Bijl, de Graaf, *et al.*, 2001).

The terms 'social networks' and 'connectedness' (or connections) were also used. Networks refer to having contact with people through the neighbourhood and community, via family and friends, or work. Connectedness is about being and feeling connected to other people. Even if there people around, you may not feel connected to them. Feeling connected to others contributes toward a sense of belonging, and loneliness is a form of disconnectedness (Holmes and Holmes, 1993).

Nurturing relationships with acquaintances, friends, or family is worthwhile. There is evidence that befriending programs, which link volunteers with individuals who are depressed, can be effective (Harris, Brown, and Robinson, 1999). Relationships can be fostered by keeping in contact, being interested in what the other person is doing, and helping each other out. Sometimes there are rifts in families or with friends. These may be able to be mended, though sometimes they cannot.

If there is a problem in a relationship, you may want to look at options for dealing with the problem. Talking with friends or a relationship counsellor about it, or working through the problem-solving steps outlined in Step 4, may help you identify possible solutions. (See the later discussion in this step about resolving conflict.)

The importance of activity was highlighted in the last step, and involvement in social activities was encouraged. By getting involved in the neighbourhood or community, good links can be made with local people. Taking a course, or joining a club or support group may be helpful too.

One of the benefits of becoming more involved socially is that we tend to focus less on ourselves and our concerns. This can be a healthy thing at times. Being alone at times and feeling comfortable with that is also very healthy.

DEVELOPING ASSERTIVENESS

The who, what, why, how, when and where of assertiveness!

Who needs to be assertive?

We all need to be able to express ourselves assertively or directly at times. Do you have difficulty expressing your opinion, or find it hard to be clear in what you want to say? Do you find your needs are not being met, or that you unintentionally upset people with what you say? If the answer is yes to any of these questions, then working on becoming more assertive is important for you (Page and Page, 1996; WHO, 1997). In the long run being more assertive also helps develop a greater sense of self-esteem.

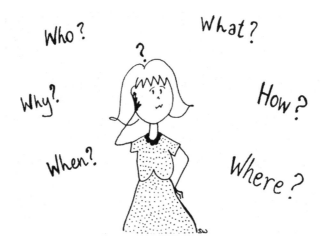

What is assertiveness?

Assertiveness means **being able to express your needs and feelings more directly**. It involves changing the ways in which you relate to people and the behaviours that you use (Corey, 2008).

What can you gain from being more assertive? It can be helpful in starting conversations, confronting others, dealing with annoyance, responding to criticism, turning down requests or asking for favours (WHO, 1997).

Assertiveness is based on a number of rules and rights (Williams, 2000). These are worth remembering.

'**I have the right to . . .**'

➤ respect myself

➤ recognise my own needs as an individual
➤ make clear 'I' statements
➤ allow myself to make mistakes
➤ change my mind
➤ ask for 'thinking-over time'
➤ allow myself to enjoy my successes
➤ ask for what I want
➤ recognise that I am not responsible for the behaviour of other adults
➤ respect other people.

The table below summarises three different types of behaviours. There is passive behaviour, which is the opposite of assertive behaviour, and there is aggressive behaviour, which is quite different from assertiveness (Page and Page, 1996).

PASSIVE	AGGRESSIVE	ASSERTIVE
Do you . . .	Do you . . .	Do you . . .
avoid saying what you think or feel?	tend to offend others when you stand up for yourself or for your rights?	clearly communicate your feelings, thoughts and needs to others?
avoid telling people what you want or would like?	struggle to communicate effectively?	avoid saying it doesn't matter when it does, in a tactful way?
put other people's needs before your own?	wait until you are really frustrated about something and then 'explode'?	respect your own rights, but also those of others?
feel as if you are weak, inferior or incompetent?	talk over others and not let them have their say?	

(Page and Page, 1996; World Health Organization Collaborating Centre for Mental Health and Substance Abuse, 2000)

There are different types of assertion (Page and Page, 1996). There is positive assertion (giving compliments), and there is negative assertion, such as refusing a request or saying 'No'. Here is an example of negative assertion: you are getting ready to go out for dinner when a friend rings and asks if you can baby-sit her child.
➤ The passive response would be to say 'Yes.'
➤ The aggressive response would be to say 'You can't ask me to put myself out like that.'
➤ An assertive response would be 'Unfortunately I can't help right now – I already have a commitment.'

Why does non-assertiveness develop?
Assertive and non-assertive behaviours are learned. As a child we are taught how to behave. For example, how did your family handle conflict? What did they do when they disagreed with someone? What did you learn from them? In what ways

did you learn to get what you wanted without asking for it directly, for example, by yelling or crying? Do you still use those ways? (WHO, 1997)

There can be obstacles to being assertive, such as fear of offending the other person, or worry that they won't approve. It is good to be sensitive to others, but your rights are important too, and you are not responsible for how the other person reacts (Page and Page, 1996). Being more assertive can impact on relationships. Those around you can be used to interacting with you in certain ways, and may feel challenged when you become more assertive. It is important to be aware of this.

Look back at the role of beliefs in our thinking (Step 5). A belief in needing approval from everyone can be a barrier to being assertive. Shyness or a problem with social anxiety (Step 1) can also be a barrier to speaking out.

How to be more assertive
Firstly, what do you say? It is helpful to use 'I' statements. These can explain:
1. your feelings about the person's behaviour or the effect of the behaviour ('I feel . . .')
2. what the unacceptable behaviour is in a non-blameful way ('When you . . .')
3. the effects of the behaviour on you ('Because . . .')
4. what you want to happen ('I'd prefer . . .')

(Burns, 1992; O'Connor, 2001).

It is important to also acknowledge the other person at the start of what you say. This means saying something like 'I appreciate . . .' or 'I can see that you feel . . .'

Here is an example.

'I can see that you are feeling annoyed. However, I feel upset when you tell me I'm hopeless, because it affects my confidence. I want you to stop saying that and recognise that I do a lot of things well.'

Secondly, how does being assertive look and sound? Here are some tips:
➤ stand or sit firmly, and be upright and not fidgeting
➤ have an open body posture (no folded arms or crossed legs)
➤ speak in a clear steady tone of voice, in a calm way
➤ use eye contact, and have relaxed facial features.

The key is to **practise**. Practise with your GP, MHP or with a friend, or in front of the mirror. Even write scripts to help practise what you want to say (Gressor, 1996).

Identify situations where you might need to be assertive and prepare for them. If you have to speak with someone over the phone, for example, you could make some notes and have them in front of you.

Here are a few more tips on how, when and where to put assertiveness into practice.

There are some situations in which it is very difficult to be assertive, for example, if the other person is being aggressive. It may help to:

➤ repeat your answer
➤ not respond to inappropriate conversation or requests
➤ refuse to carry on a conversation with that person until the anger dies down.

Here is another example: you are in a conversation where the other person is mixing up issues and raising unrelated emotional issues. You could say 'It's not that I don't care about that issue, but I don't want to discuss it at the moment. I want to focus on . . .'

Feelings of guilt can get in the way of assertiveness. You may like to do a really good or perfect job, and others may try to get what they want by making you feel guilty. Be aware of this if you are prone to guilt. Remember that sorry is a word that we can overuse – only say 'sorry' if it is genuine.

Practise saying 'No'. Remind yourself of why you are saying no – that you don't have the time, it's inconvenient, or you are not interested – and be direct about it.

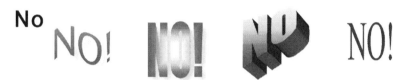

Use tact when you are making requests, as this allows the other person to say yes or no. Be specific and give the reasons as to why you are asking them to do something, for example, 'I'm tired . . .' Don't wait until the last minute (WHO, 1997).

DEALING WITH RELATIONSHIP ISSUES

Relationships are a central part of life. Dealing with relationship issues can be an important part of managing depression. A relationship breakdown may have contributed to the development of depression. Relationship problems may be causing ongoing stress – perhaps there are problems in communicating, or bullying or domestic violence in a relationship.

Often there are issues around intimacy with a partner. Depression itself can lower libido, and medication can sometimes have a negative effect. Low energy levels, ongoing stress and tiredness can also be barriers to enjoying a sexual relationship. Talk with your GP or MHP if you have sexual concerns as they may be able to make some suggestions.

Whatever the issues, relationships often need some help. You may be able to do some work on this yourself – or it may be appropriate to ask for help from your GP or MHP. Getting a referral for expert relationship counselling may be useful.

All relationships need to be looked after and nourished. Time and effort are important. So is being interested in the other person, having a positive attitude and not criticising. Listening is vital, and you can show that you are listening through being attentive and making good eye contact (Gressor, 1996). Everyone wants to be heard and understood.

Sometimes difficult situations arise in relationships. Here are a few examples.

1. There is a problem to deal with or decision to make, but neither you nor your friend / partner can work out how to deal with it. Talking with others may help, or you can try the problem-solving strategy outlined in Step 4. It can help you to find the best solution, bearing in mind that there often isn't a perfect solution.

2. You or your partner want everything to be perfect or 100% under control, or someone in a relationship thinks they know what the other person is thinking. Look back to Step 5 and the thinking errors outlined there. What thinking errors might get in the way in relationships? You can apply the same CBT principles to relationships as to an individual.

3. Someone in the relationship is very insecure, needing constant reassurance, or has jealousy issues. Perhaps low self-esteem is a factor. Look back to Step 6.

Conflict is an issue all relationships need to deal with. This involves a clash in opinions. How do you handle conflict in relationships?

_____
_____
_____
_____
_____
_____
_____
_____
_____

These are some useful questions to ask in working out how to deal with conflict.
➤ Is the conflict related to emotions or are emotions getting in the way of resolving the conflict?
➤ What are the emotions?
➤ If anger, who is angry?
➤ If mistrust, who is mistrustful?
➤ If fear, who is fearful?
➤ Is jealousy or guilt involved?
➤ What issues are underlying the conflict?
➤ What are each person's needs or wants?
➤ Could there be a misunderstanding?
➤ Is everyone taking responsibility for their actions?
➤ Are there power or control issues in the relationship?
(Scott, 1990)

There are different strategies and options for resolving conflict. You may decide to:
➤ work through the conflict by sorting out what each person wants and seeing if needs can be met
➤ look at all the possible options and choose the best possible option
➤ change your opinion (or the other person may change theirs)
➤ come to a compromise
➤ agree to differ
➤ avoid relationships where there is a strong clash.
(Gressor, 1996; Page and Page, 1996)

Many of these strategies involve sitting down and communicating about the important issues for each person, but sometimes you may need to spend time away from each other first to calm down. It can also be helpful to take turns in speaking and agree to let the other person talk or listen. You may have to talk about underlying fears and jealousies (Scott, 1990).

Here is a strategy that may help sort out conflict. It is similar to the problem-solving technique outlined in Step 4.

---

1. Name the problem – name the conflict:

2. List possible solutions:

3. Weigh up the advantages and disadvantages:

4. Choose the best possible solution:

5. Plan the steps to be taken:

6. Review the result:

Separation and divorce are associated with many challenges and stresses. They cause loss and grief, and there are often feelings of hurt and anger to be worked through. Again, it may be useful to seek counselling. Agencies such as Relationships Australia offer counselling and group courses on adjusting to separation.

The principles outlined in Step 6 on managing loss and grief are also helpful here. Look after yourself by eating properly and avoid increasing your smoking or drinking. Find ways to express your feelings constructively – talking with friends, working hard in the garden, exercising, writing in a journal. Avoid rushing into decisions. Get sound advice and take your time.

DEALING WITH UNEMPLOYMENT

Unemployment is a common problem in today's society. Being unemployed can have many adverse effects on the individual – from withdrawing from friends and family and feeling lonely, to impacting on sleep and daily routine. Self-esteem often falls, and of course there is the financial strain of being unemployed. A number of studies have explored the effects of unemployment on mental health, finding that unemployment causes increased levels of stress and hinders recovery from mental health problems (Leino-Arjas, Liira, Mutanen, *et al.*, 1999; Weich, 1998).

Again, talking with your GP or MHP about the stresses may help. Some mental health or community services have financial advisors who can assist.

It is a real trap to sleep at odd hours and become more and more inactive. Try to maintain a daily routine, and stay involved in activities. Explore whether there are community, volunteer or training programs available.

IDENTIFYING SUPPORTS

One way of identifying who or what your supports are in life is to draw a 'support map'. Family or friends, acquaintances or local people may be a support. Work, the Church, a community club or service may provide a regular social contact with people. An interest such as reading or sewing might be a 'friend' to you, or your pet.

Use the blank paper provided on the next page. Put yourself (you can use your name, or a circle or drawing to identify yourself) on that page where you choose. Around you, put the people and things that give you support in your life. Distance them from you, based on how important the relationship is; that is, the closer you put them, the more important they are to you.

(Capacchione, 1989; Martin, Clark, Beckinsale, *et al.,* 1997)

Points to remember
- Being connected to others socially is important to mental health.
- We all need to be able to express ourselves assertively.
- The key is to practise.
- Relationship issues are central, and all relationships need to deal with conflict.
- Unemployment can affect mental health.
- Identifying your social supports is useful.

NOTES PAGE

Developing a plan to manage early relapse symptoms

'We must always change, renew, rejuvenate ourselves; otherwise we harden' (Goethe)

In Step 1 the potential for depression to relapse was outlined. The terms 'relapse' and 'recurrence' of depression were explained. Relapse refers to an early return of symptoms before full recovery, while recurrence refers to return of symptoms after a time of being symptom-free (Kupfer, 1991).

The strategies utilised in this program aim to prevent both relapse and recurrence of depression. The program targets risk factors for relapse such as negative thinking patterns and lack of social support, and provides a means of developing protective factors such as improving coping skills, working on relationships and developing more optimistic thinking.

The program encourages **persistence** with antidepressant medication if this has been part of the treatment plan. The program relies on your own efforts, with guidance from your GP or MHP. It encourages you to work through the suggested strategies in a step-by-step way, and to see your GP or MHP regularly to monitor your progress.

This step in the program involves **maintaining the skills that you have learned.** What skills do you think have been most helpful?

_____
_____
_____
_____
_____
_____
_____

It is also important to maintain your general health and reduce stress. In what ways can you continue to do so in the future?

_____
_____

_____
_____
_____
_____
_____

Consider too, what things might get in the way of you using your new skills? And how can you deal with these situations? (Williams, 2000)

_____
_____
_____
_____
_____
_____

It is important to continue medication for as long as prescribed. Make sure that you are clear about how long to continue the medication. Discuss this with your GP and make a note of when you started the medication, and when it is likely that you will stop the medication.

_____
_____
_____
_____

When the time comes to stop the medication, it is important to discuss with your GP how to go about stopping. Sometimes it is better to continue medication long-term. Again, this is something that you and your GP can discuss.

THREE VITAL STEPS IN DEVELOPING A PLAN

1. The first step is to learn to **identify the early warning symptoms**. These are the early symptoms that you experience when becoming depressed. They might include difficulty sleeping, tiredness, tearfulness, loss of interest in usual activities, or increased irritability or anxiety (Hickie, Scott, Ricci, _et al._, 2000; WHO, 1997).

List your early warning symptoms of depression in the table below. Here are a few tips for identifying early warning symptoms.
➤ Think broadly, because depression can affect how you think as well as feel and behave. This includes how you relate to people. For example, you might withdraw from people (Williams, 2000; Yapko, 1997).
➤ Try to be specific in how you describe the symptom (WHO, 1997).
➤ It may be helpful to ask a friend or relative what they noticed early in the depression.

My early warning symptoms of depression

1.

2.

3.

4.

5.

[Note – you may want to advise someone close to you about these early warning symptoms. Sometimes it is easier for them to notice changes than for you (WHO, 1997).]

2. The second step is to **identify possible high-risk situations** for relapse. Each person is different. There may be times when you become stressed, or overtired. Perhaps it is relationship difficulties that increase the likelihood of relapse, or becoming less involved with certain activities (Preston, 2004). It may be that a certain time of the year, such as Christmas or the anniversary of losing someone close, is difficult.

Think about situations that might be high-risk for you, and write them down.

List of possible high–risk situations

1.

2.

3.

4.

Now consider what you need to do to protect yourself, or do differently if a situation like this occurs. You will be able to use some of the skills that you have learned during this program – for example, relaxation or problem-solving techniques.

How I can cope with high-risk situations

3. The last step is to **prepare an emergency plan** to put into action when you recognise that the depression is relapsing. This might include:
   - monitoring and challenging your thinking
   - focusing on the here and now
   - taking some time out
   - getting support from friends or family
   - making an earlier, or urgent, appointment with your GP or MHP
   - using medication (restarting or increasing the dose under the guidance of your GP)
   - talking with your GP or MHP
   - expressing how you feel
   - using problem solving
   - reviewing the earlier steps in this program.

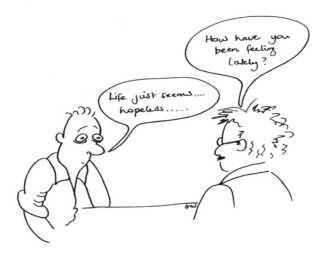

Now work on an emergency plan. Try to target your early warning symptoms, and make your plan as specific as possible (Williams, 2000). You may want to include contact numbers of people who can help you.

My emergency plan for relapse

Keep your plan in a place where you can get hold of it easily. Refer to it if needed.

Here is a summary of the steps for you to use.

My early warning symptoms of depression

1.

2.

3.

4.

5.

Possible high-risk situations for me

1.

2.

3.

4.

How to cope with high-risk situations:

My emergency plan for relapse

To finish this step, it is always good to focus on positive things. So make a note of how you know when you are improving from the depression (Yapko, 1997). Do you sleep better, cry less often, have more energy or get more done?

Signs of improvement

Points to remember
- It is important to:
  - maintain the skills that you have learned
  - maintain your general health and well-being
  - continue medication for as long as advised.
- Three vital steps in developing a plan for managing relapse are:
  - identify the early warning symptoms
  - identify possible high-risk situations
  - prepare an emergency plan.

Reassess and review, plus helpful resources

'The roots of education are bitter, but the fruit is sweet' (Aristotle)

REASSESSMENT

Well done – you have worked hard! This is the last step in the program, and there is a little more work to go. Your GP or MHP may ask you to repeat the same psychological assessments that you completed at the beginning of the program. Doing this will help you and your GP or MHP review your progress.

REVIEW OF STEPS 1–9

The 'points to remember' from each of the 10 steps are repeated here. Re-read them and consider these questions.

➤ What did you learn about yourself?
➤ What strengths did you find in yourself?
➤ What did you learn from the depression?
➤ What do you do differently now?
➤ What further steps will you take in recovering from depression and staying well?
➤ What did you find most helpful during the program?
➤ How will you persist in doing these helpful things in your life?

_____
_____
_____
_____
_____
_____
_____
_____
_____
_____

The ten-step relapse prevention program involves these steps.
1. Learning about depression and its treatment.
2. Having a check-up and setting some goals.
3. Adopting a healthy lifestyle.
4. Learning useful coping skills, such as managing stress.
5. Using helpful thinking strategies.
6. Dealing with psychological issues, such as loss or anger.
7. Becoming more active and enjoying the benefits.
8. Developing greater social support or skills.
9. Having a plan to manage early symptoms of relapse.
10. Reviewing progress, and making use of helpful resources.

STEP 1: GETTING STARTED: INFORMATION ABOUT DEPRESSION

This step contained a great deal of information about depression. It is worth having another look at the key issues. Perhaps tick what you think are the most important messages for you to hold onto.

Points to remember
➤ Understanding depression is important.
➤ Depression is common.
➤ In depression, mood is persistently and severely depressed – affecting the ability to cope and function.
➤ Depression is not weakness.
➤ It affects a person's thoughts, feelings and everyday functioning.
➤ Thought processes change in depression – there is a negative thinking and feeling cycle.
➤ Anxiety symptoms may occur or worsen.
➤ There may be biological, psychological and social factors involved in depression.
➤ Stressful life events and loss and grief may be triggers of depression.
➤ The individual is not to blame for the depression.
➤ There are risk factors for depression as well as protective factors. It is important to be aware of the risk factors and to try and minimise them, and to encourage the protective factors.
➤ There are risks from depression, including suicide, drug use and relationship breakdown.
➤ Treatment of depression is effective. It reduces risks of depression and of relapse.
➤ You will improve.
➤ Ongoing monitoring of progress is important.
➤ There is a variety of treatment strategies for addressing the bio-psychosocial needs of the individual.

➤ Treatment varies depending upon the severity and stage of the depression.
➤ Antidepressants are helpful in significant depression, especially if there are suicidal ideas.
➤ One of the most frequently used medications is SSRIs.
➤ Choice of antidepressant and dose depends on the individual.
➤ Antidepressants are effective but they take time to work.
➤ They can have side effects, but these often lessen over time.
➤ They are not addictive.
➤ PERSISTENCE is important.
➤ Please don't stop antidepressants before discussing with your GP.
➤ There is a range of talking therapies for depression, including counselling and cognitive-behavioural therapy (CBT), interpersonal therapy (IPT) and acceptance and commitment therapy (ACT).
➤ CBT has been shown to be effective in treating depression and preventing relapse.
➤ This relapse prevention program incorporates aspects of a number of different talking therapies.
➤ It aims to help you with overall functioning and well-being, by using a holistic approach.
➤ Work with your GP or MHP – they can provide information and advice, support and counselling.
➤ Gather information; write it down along with your questions.
➤ Talk with family and friends; be honest with your family and doctor.
➤ You are not alone in dealing with depression.
➤ Working through this program is a positive step.
➤ This program focuses on self-care; it helps you find your own ways to help yourself.
➤ Think about keeping a journal.
➤ In the future, keep using the skills that you have learned.
➤ Treatment takes time and it is important to persist.
➤ *Relapse* and *recurrence* refer to return of the symptoms of depression.
➤ Symptoms of anxiety and depression may be experienced at the same time. Anxiety is a distressing inner feeling of fear.
➤ This treatment program also involves strategies to help reduce symptoms of anxiety.

STEP 2: ASSESSMENT AND GOAL SETTING

Remember the importance of assessment and goal setting.
➤ **Review and rewrite your goal lists regularly**. They may change as different aspects of recovery assume more importance. For example, improving your health may be a priority at one stage, while resuming an interest or returning to work may be at another stage. As you feel able you can focus on **longer-term goals.**

➤ **Focus on your achievements** (no matter how small), and **what you have learned** from your goal setting, even if you do not reach a particular goal.

Use the sheet on goal setting provided in Step 2 to review your goals.

STEP 3: HEALTHY LIFESTYLE ISSUES

Again, there is a great deal of information in this section. Your GP or MHP will have worked with you on a 'prescription for a healthier lifestyle'. Keep that script in mind, and try to follow it through.

Points to remember

➤ Lifestyle refers to the way in which we live.
➤ Self-care is important.
➤ In depression, lifestyle changes may be needed and can be helpful.
➤ Appetite is often affected by depression.
➤ A healthy diet provides all the nutrients we need, avoids excess, and is enjoyable.
➤ Exercise has a positive effect on how you feel.
➤ Try to make exercise part of your life – slowly build up the amount that you do.
➤ Sleep can be upset in depression. Try not to worry.
➤ Keep a sleep diary, and review the tips that can help you sleep better.
➤ Stress is part of life. It means different things to different people.
➤ Stress can be triggered by external or internal factors.
➤ Stress is a three-part process with a stressor, the reaction of the mind and body, and a response.
➤ The 'fight-or-flight' response is involved.
➤ Stress can be both a positive and negative experience.
➤ Stress that persists can cause exhaustion and proneness to illness.
➤ Identifying situations which cause stress, and also factors within yourself, are important steps in managing stress.
➤ Strategies for coping with stress include problem- and emotion-focused strategies.
➤ It is important to identify how you respond to and cope with stress, and what your main concerns are underlying the stress.
➤ Don't forget general measures for dealing with stress such as keeping healthy, nurturing yourself, taking breaks and doing enjoyable activities.

You will see that a number of messages were repeated in Steps 2 and 3. Which ones are particularly important to you?

_____
_____
_____
_____

_____

_____
_____
_____

STEP 4: USEFUL COPING SKILLS

This step included a number of practical skills. Continue to work on putting them into practice, and go back to them as you need to.

Points to remember

➤ It is useful to keep a diary of your mood.

➤ As things improve, try to focus on positive feelings and thoughts.

➤ Problem solving is a useful practical strategy. It involves sorting out what the problems are and looking at logical, practical ways of dealing with each of them.

➤ There can be a lethargy cycle in depression. Self-defeating thoughts, feelings and actions can be linked.

➤ Perfectionists often defeat themselves by setting unattainably high standards.

➤ Activity brightens mood. Daily activity scheduling is another practical strategy to restore some normality in life.

➤ There are physical and mental benefits from relaxing.

➤ Everyone can gain benefits from learning to relax more.

➤ Enjoy physical relaxation, breathing techniques and visualisation.

➤ Other relaxation ideas include meditation, yoga and tai chi.

➤ Hypnotherapy can be valuable in learning how to relax.

➤ Simply enjoying your garden or walking can be relaxing.

➤ A panic attack is a discrete episode of intense fear or discomfort.

➤ Treatment involves education, explanation and reassurance that panic is not dangerous.

➤ Coping strategies include breathing, learning how to deal with situations in which panic occurs, and challenging negative thinking.

➤ Use relaxation techniques, don't rush, and take care of yourself.

➤ Deal with underlying causes of anxiety, and use what has helped in the past.

STEP 5: HELPFUL THINKING OR COGNITIVE STRATEGIES

This step is a really important one to understand and put into practice. The more that you apply the CBT strategies you've learned, the more benefit you will feel. One of the risk factors for relapse of depression is said to be persisting negative styles of thinking (Evans, Burrows and Norman, 2000). CBT can help you develop a more helpful thinking style.

Points to remember

➤ CBT is a useful and effective way to tackle symptoms of anxiety and depression.

➤ The way we think affects how we feel.
➤ Automatic thoughts may be positive or negative.
➤ Follow the five steps to tackle the unhelpful thinking that can occur in depression:
  • keeping a thought diary
  • understanding thinking errors
  • identifying thinking errors
  • challenging unhelpful thinking
  • developing more helpful thoughts.

Reflect on mindfulness and ACT.

What coping skills or helpful thinking strategies have you developed? What more can you work on?

_____
_____
_____
_____
_____
_____

STEP 6: DEALING WITH PSYCHOLOGICAL ISSUES

This step is one of the keys to healing and recovery from depression, and remaining well. Remember that we continue to learn about ourselves and develop throughout life.

Self-esteem

➤ One of the most important tasks in dealing with depression is improving self-esteem – how you see and judge yourself.
➤ Early life experiences can affect self-esteem.
➤ Our worth is not solely about what we achieve.
➤ What is really important is what you think about yourself.
➤ We need to be realistic and flexible, and practise patience and acceptance in life.

To improve self-esteem:
  1. use CBT techniques
  2. recognise your positives and reassess your negatives
  3. remember that each individual is special and unique
  4. let go of the things you don't like about yourself, and learn from mistakes
  5. develop your strengths
  6. self-respect is important
  7. develop creativity
  8. aim for self-acceptance and love.

Loss and grief
➤ Adjusting to loss and grief takes time.
➤ It is important to understand the process of grief, and share thoughts and feelings about the loss.
➤ Allow 'grief time' each day.
➤ Look after yourself; take time out.
➤ If possible, find some meaning out of the loss.
➤ Challenge unhelpful thinking related to the grief.
➤ Self-esteem can be affected in grief.
➤ Achieving a sense of closure is important.

The 'negative' emotions
➤ We all experience a range of emotions – anger, guilt, shame, jealousy and hate.
➤ Anger is what you feel when provoked, and can be a normal response to many situations.
➤ Anger-management skills can be important.
➤ Work on understanding and dealing with the thinking associated with the anger, jealousy, guilt or shame.
➤ Work out how much responsibility *you* need to take and how much others are responsible for.

Letting go, loneliness and hopelessness
➤ Good communication with others is important.
➤ Letting go of negative emotions can be very valuable.
➤ Focus on enriching your life and connecting with others.
➤ If feeling suicidal, talk with your GP. Remember that you are not alone – there are solutions to problems and help is available.
➤ Hope is vital.
➤ There are different ways to think about and explore meaning and purpose in life.
➤ Recognise the things that you can be thankful for.
➤ Inspirational writing can be very encouraging.

STEP 7: THE BENEFITS OF ACTIVITY
Some vital points were highlighted in this step.

Points to remember
➤ Activity is central to life.
➤ Depression can be helped by activity.
➤ Give yourself permission to enjoy different activities.
➤ Include pleasurable activities in your day.
➤ Keep life simple.
➤ Smile and laugh.
➤ Develop your compassion, enjoy giving.

STEP 8: FOSTERING SOCIAL SUPPORT AND SKILLS

➤ Having social connections is important to mental health.
➤ We all need to be able to express ourselves assertively.
➤ The key is to practise.
➤ Relationship issues are central, and all relationships need to deal with conflict.
➤ Unemployment can affect mental health.
➤ Identifying your social supports is useful.

What activities or social situations do you enjoy? How can you become more involved in these?

_____
_____
_____
_____
_____

STEP 9: DEVELOPING A PLAN TO MANAGE EARLY SYMPTOMS OF RELAPSE

It is important to:
➤ maintain the skills that you have learned
➤ maintain your general health and well-being
➤ continue medication for as long as advised.

Three vital steps in developing a plan for managing relapse are:
1. identify the early warning symptoms
2. identify possible high-risk situations
3. prepare an emergency plan.

Remind yourself about your emergency plan.

My emergency plan for relapse

CONCLUSION

There is a meditation based on the work of Pelletier (cited in Hammond, 1990) which begins with imagining a beautiful tree – with strong roots, a broad trunk and leafy branches spreading upward. The meditation acknowledges the strength and beauty of the tree, and how it is in balance with nature – taking what it needs to grow and survive, and giving back – through making oxygen, giving shelter or producing fruit.

The meditation moves on to contemplating oneself – having strengths like the tree, giving and taking, but being able to speak, move and love as well. We can see the wonder of the tree, and the meditation invites us to look at ourselves in a positive way too, and recognise our own strengths and abilities (Pelletier, cited in Hammond, 1990).

On the following page you will find a drawing of a tree that you can use to make some notes.

➤ In the ground below the tree, where the roots are, name some of your strengths?
➤ Around the trunk write some of your supports.
➤ In the area of the leaves and branches name what you are aiming for, and what you consider to be important in life.

Take time to do this task – even ask a family member or friend for help if you want to. Many of the resources are within you – and around you.

This program was developed with the aim of helping you to recover from the depression and to stay well in the future. It has looked at the physical, psychological, social and spiritual aspect of your mental health.

Well done for working through the program. You and your GP or MHP will continue to work together. Keep looking after yourself, focus on the positive gains that you are making and continue to develop your own resources and resilience. In doing so you will be 'keeping the blues away'.

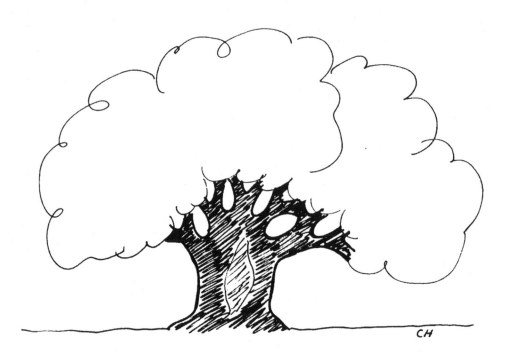

Resources: Where to go for help

BOOKS
Books on depression

Aisbett B. *Taming the Black Dog: a guide to overcoming depression.* Pymble, NSW: Harper Collins; 2000.

A helpful and very readable book, incorporating a cognitive approach. It has amusing cartoons and is particularly liked by young people.

Golant M, Golant S. *What to Do When Someone You Love is Depressed: a practical, compassionate, and helpful guide.* New York, NY: Henry Holt and Co; 1996.

A useful book for friends and relatives to read. It explains depression, its impact on relationships, and how to support the person with depression as well as look after oneself.

Kidman A. *Feeling Better: a guide to mood management.* 2nd ed. St Leonards, NSW: Biochemical & General Services; 2006.

This wise book has many useful charts and tips.

Preston J. *You Can Beat Depression: a guide to prevention and recovery.* 4th ed. Atascadero, CA: Impact Publishers; 2004.

A very readable book, with good sections on the causes of depression and relapse prevention.

Tanner S, Ball J. *Beating the Blues: a self-help approach to overcoming depression.* Sydney, NSW: Doubleday; 2001.

An excellent book explaining the cognitive approach to treating depression. There is a chapter about depression written for the family.

Wolpert L. *Malignant Sadness: the anatomy of depression.* London, UK: Faber & Faber; 1999.

Lewis Wolpert is a Professor of Biology. He writes about his own experiences with depression. Some people really relate to this account of depression.

Books on anxiety

Aisbett B. *Living With It: a survivor's guide to panic attacks.* Sydney, NSW: Angus & Robertson; 1993.

Another good little book by this author, based on cognitive therapy. A seemingly light-hearted approach to panic attacks, but full of gems of wisdom. Most people find this a really useful book.

Fox B. *Power Over Panic: freedom from panic/anxiety related disorders.* Frenchs Forest, NSW: Longman; 1996.
A very readable book on anxiety and panic, using case histories to illustrate important points.

Marks I. *Living With Fear: understanding and coping with anxiety.* Maidenhead, UK: McGraw Hill; 2005.
A gold standard book on anxiety. More lengthy, but a good read if you want more detailed information.

Books on cognitive therapy

Burns D. *Feeling Good: the new mood therapy.* New York, NY: Avon Books Inc.; 1999.
Explains cognitive therapy for depression. Quite detailed, but has sections that apply to the individual that can be focused on.

Burns D. *The Feeling Good Handbook.* New York, NY: Plume; 1999.
The self-help guide that accompanies 'Feeling Good: the new mood therapy'. Lengthy.

Edelman S. *Change Your Thinking.* 2nd ed. Sydney, NSW: ABC Books. 2006.
This book is easy to understand and helps the reader apply the principles of cognitive therapy to difficult situations.

Greenberger D, Padesky C. *Mind Over Mood: change how you feel by changing the way you think.* New York, NY: The Guilford Press; 1995.
A clearly set out, practical book with exercises to be completed.

Padesky C, Greenberger D. *Clinician's Guide to Mind Over Mood.* New York, NY: The Guilford Press; 1995.
A guide for clinicians to use in helping patients work through 'Mind Over Mood'.

Tanner S, Ball J. *Beating the Blues: a self-help approach to overcoming depression.* Sydney, NSW: Doubleday; 2001.
An excellent guide to CBT in depression.

Books on acceptance and commitment therapy

Harris R. *The Happiness Trap: stop struggling, start living.* Wollombi, NSW: Exisle Publishing; 2007.
An excellent book on ACT, easy to read and many creative ideas.

Books on lifestyle

A range of lifestyle issues are well covered in the books cited below:

Brand-Miller J, Foster-Powell K. *The Glucose Revolution: G.I. plus.* Sydney, NSW: Hodder Mobius; 2000.

Carlson R. *Don't Sweat the Small Stuff:. . . and it's all small stuff.* New York, NY: Hyperion; 1977.

Clifton P, Noakes M. *The CSIRO Total Well-Being Diet.* Camberwell, Vic: Penguin; 2005.

Garth M. *The Inner Garden: meditations for life from 9 to 90.* Melbourne, Vic: Collins Dove; 1994.

Holden R. *Laughter the Best Medicine: the healing powers of happiness, humour and joy.* New York, NY: Thorsons; 1993.

Hopkins C. *101 Shortcuts to Relaxation.* London, UK: Bloomsbury; 1997.

Michie D. *Hurry Up and Meditate.* Sydney, NSW: Allen & Unwin; 2008.

Wilson Schaef A. *Meditations for Living in Balance: daily solutions for people who do too much.* New York, NY: Harper Collins; 2000.

Wilson P. *Instant Calm: over 100 easy-to-use techniques for relaxing mind and body.* Ringwood, Vic: Penguin; 1995.

WEBSITES
Australian
Keeping the blues away: www.keepingthebluesaway.com

Beyondblue: www.beyondblue.org.au

Blue pages: www.bluepages.anu.edu.au

MoodGym: http://moodgym.anu.edu.au

DepressioNET: www.depressionservices.org.au

Grow: www.grow.net.au/igrow

Blackdog Institute: www.blackdoginstitute.org.au

Department of Health and Ageing on mental health and wellbeing: www.health.gov.au/internet/main/publishing.nsf/Content/portal-Mental%20health

Royal Australian and New Zealand College of Psychiatrists: www.ranzcp.org/

Clinical Research Unit for Anxiety Disorders – information on diagnosis and treatment for consumers and professionals: www.crufad.com

Panic and Anxiety Hub – helping people learn about anxiety: www.paems.com.au

SANE Australia: www.sane.org/

Patient information sheets on depression and anxiety by Professor John Murtagh: www.nevdgp.org.au/info/murtagh/general/index.htm

For young people
Headroom: www.headroom.net.au

beyondblue website for young people: www.ybblue.com.au

SANE website for young people: www.itsallright.org

Centre for Adolescent Health: www.rch.org.au/cah

Reachout website: www.reachout.com.au

About grief
Grieflink: www.grieflink.org.au

Centre for Grief Education: www.grief.org.au

About lifestyle issues
Department of Health and Ageing on nutrition and physical activity: www.health.gov.au/internet/main/publishing.nsf/Content/Nutrition+and+Physical+Activity-1

Mind Body Life: www.mindbodylife.com.au/

'Sleep Better Without Drugs' program information: www.sleepbetter.com.au

British

Royal College of Psychiatrists in the United Kingdom – user-friendly information about mental health problems: www.rcpsych.ac.uk/public/help/welcome.htm

World Health Organization – useful mental health information: www.whoguidemhpcuk.org/

The Happiness Project: www.happiness.co.uk

International Stress Management Association: www.isma.org.uk

American

For GP information and depression guidelines: www.mentalhealth.com

www.surgeongeneral.gov/library/mentalhealth

Stress Release Health Enterprises – information about anxiety and panic: www.stress release.com

COMMUNITY RESOURCES

SANE Helpline (information and referral regarding mental health problems): 1800 688 382

beyondblue info line: 1300 22 4636

Kids Help Line: 1800 55 1800

GROW Community Centres: 1800 558 268

Relationships Australia (bookshop, library and courses): 02 6285 4466 (National office)

Community Health Centres: listed in phonebook

Local libraries: listed in phonebook

Make a list of your local community resources here

TREATMENT SERVICES

➤ Your local GP.

➤ Your local community health centres.

➤ Community mental health teams of the State Mental Health Services.

➤ To find out more about private psychologists, psychiatrists, or qualified hypnotherapists the following organisations can be contacted:

- The Australian Psychological Society: 1800 333 497
- Royal Australian and New Zealand College of Psychiatrists: 1800 337 448
- Australian Society of Hypnosis: State branch contact details can be obtained from www.ozhypnosis.com.au/state.htm

Emergency numbers

Lifeline: 13 1114

Mental Health 24-hour Emergency: 1800 182 232

Alcohol and Drug Information Service: 1300 131 340

Kids Help Line: 1800 55 1800

Other:

References

INTRODUCTION FOR CLINICIANS

Blackburn I, Davidson K. *Cognitive Therapy for Depression and Anxiety: a practitioner's guide.* 2nd ed. Oxford, UK: Blackwell Scientific Publications; 1995.

Davies J. *A Manual of Mental Health Care in General Practice.* Canberra, ACT: Commonwealth Department of Health and Aged Care; 2000.

Ellis P, The Royal Australian and New Zealand College of Psychiatrists Clinical Practice Guidelines Team for Depression. Australian and New Zealand clinical practice guidelines for the treatment of depression. *Aust NZ J Psychiatry.* 2004; **38**: 389–407.

Fava G, Rafanelli C, Grandi S, *et al.* Prevention of recurrent depression with cognitive behavioural therapy: preliminary findings. *Arch Gen Psychiatry.* 1998; **55**: 816–20.

Greenberger D, Padesky C. *Clinician's Guide to Mind Over Mood.* New York, NY: The Guilford Press; 1995.

Harris R. *The Happiness Trap: stop struggling, start living.* Wollombi, NSW: Exisle Publishing; 2007.

Hickie I. An approach to managing depression in general practice. *Med J Aust.* 2000; **173**: 106–10.

Howell, CA. Preventing depression relapse: a primary care approach. *Prim Care Ment Health.* 2004; **2**: 151–6.

Howell C, Marshall C, Opolski M, *et al.* Management of recurrent depression. *Aust Fam Physician.* 2008; **37**: 704–8.

Howell C, Turnbull D, Beilby J, *et al.* Preventing relapse of depression in primary care: a pilot study of the 'Keeping the Blues Away' program. *Med J Aust.* 2008; **188**(12 Suppl.): S138–41.

Jarrett R, Kraft D, Doyle J, *et al.* Preventing recurrent depression using cognitive therapy with and without a continuation phase: a randomised clinical trial. *Arch Gen Psychiatry.* 2001; **58**: 381–8.

Kidman A. *Feeling Better: a guide to mood management.* 2nd ed. St Leonards, NSW: Biochemical & General Services; 2006.

Paykel E, Scott J, Teasdale J, *et al.* Prevention of relapse in residual depression by cognitive therapy: a controlled trial. *Arch Gen Psychiatry.* 1999; **56**: 829–35.

Sadock BJ, Sadock VA. *Kaplan and Sadock's Synopsis of Psychiatry: behavioural sciences/clinical psychiatry.* 10th ed. Baltimore, MD: Williams and Wilkins; 2007.

Segal Z, Williams J, Teasdale J. *Mindfulness-Based Cognitive Therapy for Depression: a new approach to preventing relapse*. New York, NY: The Guilford Press; 2002.

Teasdale J, Segal Z, Williams J, *et al*. Prevention of relapse/recurrence in major depression by mindfulness-based cognitive therapy. *J Consult Clin Psychol*. 2000; **68**: 615–23.

Williams C. *Planning for the Future: a 5 areas approach*. Leeds, UK: University of Leeds Innovations; 2000.

World Health Organization (WHO) Collaborating Centre for Mental Health and Substance Abuse. *Management of Mental Disorders: treatment protocol project*. 3rd ed. Vol. 1. Sydney, NSW: Wild & Woolley; 2000.

STEP 1

Agency for Health Care Policy and Research. *Depression is a Treatable Illness: a patient's guide*. Silver Spring, MD: AHCPR Publications Clearinghouse; 1993.

American Psychiatric Association. *Diagnostic and Statistical Manual of Mental Disorders (DSM-IV-TR)*. Washington, DC: American Psychiatric Association; 2000.

Beyondblue website. www.beyondblue.org.au

Beyondblue. *Young people, alcohol and depression: a risky business* [Letter]. 2007. Available at: www.beyondblue.org.au/index.aspx?link_id=105.898&fid=925&oid=886 (accessed 27 July 2009).

Bloch S, Singh B. *Understanding Troubled Minds: a guide to mental illness and its treatment*. Melbourne, Vic: Melbourne University Press; 1997.

Braddon J, Edwards S, Warrick T, *et al*. *DATIS Review of Management of Depression in General Practice*. Adelaide, SA: Drugs and Therapeutics Information Service; 2007.

Davies J. *A Manual of Mental Health Care in General Practice*. Canberra, ACT: Commonwealth Department of Health and Aged Care; 2000.

Dryden W, Mytton J. *Four Approaches to Counselling and Psychotherapy*. London, UK: Routledge; 1999.

Ellis P, Smith D. Treating depression: the beyondblue guidelines for treating depression in primary care. *Med J Aust*. 2002; **176**(Suppl.): S77–83.

Engel G. The clinical application of the bio-psychosocial model. *Am J Psychiatry*. 1980; **137**: 535–44.

Evans B, Burrows G, Norman T. *Understanding Depression*. Kew, Vic: Mental Health Promotion Unit; 2000.

Evans B, Coman G, Burrows G. *Your Guide to Understanding and Managing Stress*. Kew, Vic: Mental Health Foundation of Victoria; 1998.

Fava G, Rafanelli C, Grandi S, *et al*. Six-year outcome for cognitive behavioural treatment of residual symptoms in major depression. *Am J Psychiatry*. 1998; **155**: 1443–5.

Fava G, Rafanelli C, Cazzaro M, *et al*. Well-being therapy: a novel psychotherapeutic approach for residual symptoms of affective disorders. *Psychol Med*. 1998; **28**: 475–80.

Fava G, Ruini C, Mangelli L. Patients with depression can be taught how to improve recovery. *BMJ*. 2001; **322**: 1428.

Gloaguen V, Cottraux J, Cucherat M, *et al*. A meta-analysis of the effects of cognitive therapy in depressed patients. *J Affect Disord*. 1998; **49**: 59–72.

Harris R. Embracing your demons: an overview of acceptance and commitment therapy. *Psychother Aust.* 2006; **12**(4): 2–8.

Harris R. *The Happiness Trap: stop struggling, start living.* Wollombi, NSW: Exisle Publishing; 2007.

Hickie I. Responding to the Australian experience of depression. *Med J Aust.* 2002; **176**(Suppl.): S61–2.

Hickie I, Andrews G, Davenport T. Measuring outcomes in patients with depression or anxiety: an essential part of clinical practice. *Med J Aust.* 2002; **177**: 205–7.

Hickie I, Scott E, Ricci C, *et al. A Depression Management Program: incorporating cognitive-behavioural strategies.* Melbourne, Vic: Educational Health Solutions; 2000.

Huibers M, Beurskens A, Bleijenberg G, *et al.* The effectiveness of psychosocial interventions delivered by general practitioners. *Cochrane Database Syst Rev.* 2003; **2**: CD003494.

Kessler R, Berglund P, Demler O, *et al.* The epidemiology of major depressive disorder: results from the National Comorbidity Survey Replication. *JAMA.* 2003; **289**: 3095–105.

Kidman A. *Feeling Better: a guide to mood management.* 2nd ed. St Leonards, NSW: Biochemical & General Services; 2006.

Koppe H. Well-being: part 1 – what is it? *Aust Fam Physician.* 2002; **31**: 374–5.

Kupfer D. Long-term treatment of depression. *J Clin Psychiatry.* 1991; **52**(Suppl.): S28–34.

Murtagh J. *Depression.* 1995. Available at: www.nevdgp.org.au/info/murtagh/general/Depression.htm (accessed 27 July 2009).

New Zealand National Health Committee. *Guidelines for the treatment and management of depression by primary healthcare professionals.* 1996. Available at: www.nzgg.org.nz/guidelines/0039/depression_guideline.pdf (accessed 27 July 2009).

Pirkis J, Stokes D, Morley B, *et al.* Impact of Australia's better outcomes in mental health care program on psychologists. *Aust Psychol.* 2006; **41**: 152–9.

Preston J. *You Can Beat Depression: a guide to prevention and recovery.* 4th ed. Atascadero, CA: Impact Publishers; 2004.

Royal Australian and New Zealand College of Psychiatrists website. www.ranzcp.org/

Royal College of Psychiatrists website. www.rcpsych.ac.uk

Sadock BJ, Sadock VA. *Kaplan and Sadock's Synopsis of Psychiatry: behavioural sciences/clinical psychiatry.* 10th ed. Baltimore, MD: Williams and Wilkins; 2007.

Segal Z, Williams J, Teasdale J. *Mindfulness-Based Cognitive Therapy for Depression: a new approach to preventing relapse.* New York, NY: The Guilford Press; 2002.

The Options Project. *Depression: causes and treatment* [pamphlet]. Victoria: Mental Health Foundation of Australia. Available at: www.embracethefuture.org.au/youth/pdf/Depression.pdf (accessed 27 July 2009).

Therapeutic Guidelines Limited. *Therapeutic guidelines: psychotropic (version 6).* 2008. Available at: www.tg.org.au/index.php?sectionid=48 (accessed 27 July 2009).

White C, Denborough D. *Introducing Narrative Therapy: a collection of practice-based writings.* Adelaide, SA: Dulwich Centre Publications; 1998.

Williams C. *Understanding and Using Antidepressant Medication: a 5 areas approach.* Leeds, UK: University of Leeds Innovations; 2000.

World Health Organization (WHO) Collaborating Centre for Mental Health and Substance Abuse. *Management of Mental Disorders: treatment protocol project.* 3rd ed. Vol. 1. Sydney, NSW: Wild & Woolley; 2000.

STEP 2

Harris R. Embracing your demons: an overview of acceptance and commitment therapy. *Psychother Aust.* 2006; 12(4): 2–8.

Harris R. *The Happiness Trap: stop struggling, start living.* Wollombi, NSW: Exisle Publishing; 2007.

Kidman A. *Feeling Better: a guide to mood management.* 2nd ed. St Leonards, NSW: Biochemical & General Services; 2006.

Sadock BJ, Sadock VA. *Kaplan and Sadock's Synopsis of Psychiatry: behavioural sciences/clinical psychiatry.* 10th ed. Baltimore, MD: Williams and Wilkins; 2007.

World Health Organization (WHO) Collaborating Centre for Mental Health and Substance Abuse. *Management of Mental Disorders: treatment protocol project.* 3rd ed. Vol. 1. Sydney, NSW: Wild & Woolley; 2000.

STEP 3

Benson H. *The Relaxation Response.* London, UK: Fountain Paperbacks; 1977.

Brand-Miller J, Foster-Powell K. *The Glucose Revolution: G.I. plus.* Sydney, NSW: Hodder Mobius; 2000.

Burns R. *10 Skills for Working with Stress.* Chatswood, NSW: Business & Professional Publishers; 1992.

CSIRO. *Fish oils keep the heart running smoothly* [fact sheet]. 2007. Available at: www.csiro.au/resources/Omega-3-fish-oils.html (accessed 27 July 2009).

Department of Health and Ageing. *Food for health: dietary guidelines for Australians.* 2005. Available at: www.nhmrc.gov.au/publications/synopses/dietsyn.htm (accessed 27 July 2009).

Evans B, Burrows G, Norman T. *Understanding Depression.* Kew, Vic: Mental Health Promotion Unit; 2000.

Evans B, Coman G, Burrows G. *Your Guide to Understanding and Managing Stress.* Kew, Vic: Mental Health Foundation of Victoria; 1998.

Evans L, Wagon R. Stress in the workplace. *Curr Ther.* 2002; 43(9): 14–16.

Gressor M, editor. *How to Stop Worrying and be Happy: coping strategies for stress, depression, grief and other common problems in the age of anxiety.* Sydney, NSW: Gore & Osment; 1996.

Hassed C. Meditation in general practice. *Aust Fam Physician.* 1996; 25: 1257–60.

Lawlor D, Hopker S. The effectiveness of exercise as an intervention in the management of depression: systematic review and meta-regression analysis of randomised clinical trials. *BMJ.* 2001; 322: 763–7.

Mori T, Bao D, Burke V, *et al.* Dietary fish as a major component of a weight-loss diet: effect on serum lipids, glucose, and insulin metabolism in overweight hypertensive subjects. *Am J Clin Nutr.* 1999; 70: 817–25.

New Zealand National Health Committee. *Guidelines for the treatment and management of depression by primary healthcare professionals.* 1996. Available at: www.nzgg.org.nz/guidelines/0039/depression_guideline.pdf (accessed 27 July 2009).

Rankin-Box D, editor. *The Nurses' Handbook of Complementary Therapies.* 2nd ed. London, UK: Bailliere Tindall; 2001.

Royal College of Psychiatrists. *Sleeping well.* 2009. Available at: www.rcpsych.ac.uk/mentalhealthinfoforall/problems/sleepproblems/sleepingwell.aspx (accessed 27 July 2009).

Singh H. Introducing stress management into general practice. *Aust Fam Physician.* 1996; **25**: 1228–31.

Stern T, Herman J, Slavin P, editors. *MGH Guide to Psychiatry in Primary Care.* New York, NY: McGraw-Hill; 1998.

Wheatley D. The role of stress in psychiatric disorders. *Int J Psychiatry Clin Pract.* 2000; **6**: 93–100.

White R. Insomnia: management in general practice. *Mod Med Aust.* 1998; **June**: 86–95.

Wilson P. *Instant Calm.* Ringwood, Vic: Penguin; 1995.

STEP 4

Aisbett B. *Living With It: a survivor's guide to panic attacks.* Sydney, NSW: Angus & Robertson; 1993.

Andrews G, Hunt C. Treatments that work in anxiety disorders. *MJA Practice Essentials Mental Health.* 1998; **5**: 26–32.

Barlow D, Craske M. *Mastery of Your Anxiety and Panic.* 4th ed. New York, NY: Oxford University Press; 2006.

Barlow J, Ellard D, Hainsworth JM, *et al.* A review of self-management interventions for panic disorders, phobias and obsessive-compulsive disorders. *Acta Psychiatr Scand.* 2005; **111**: 272–85.

Burns D. *Feeling Good: the new mood therapy.* New York, NY: Avon Books Inc.; 1999.

Corey G. *Theory and Practice of Counselling and Psychotherapy.* 8th ed. Pacific Grove, CA: Brooks & Cole; 2008.

Davies J. *A Manual of Mental Health Care in General Practice.* Canberra, ACT: Commonwealth Department of Health and Aged Care; 2000.

Fox B. *Power Over Panic: freedom from panic/anxiety related disorders.* Melbourne, Vic: Longman; 1996.

Ham M, Waters D, Oliver M. Treatment of panic disorder. *Am Fam Physician.* 2005; **71**: 733–9.

Hassed C. Meditation in general practice. *Aust Fam Physician.* 1996; **25**: 1257–60.

Hickie I, Scott E, Ricci C, *et al.* *A Depression Management Program: incorporating cognitive-behavioural strategies.* Melbourne, Vic: Educational Health Solutions; 2000.

Hunter M. *Daydreams for Discovery: a manual for hypnotherapists.* West Vancouver, Canada: Sea Walk Press; 1988.

Kidman A. *Feeling Better: a guide to mood management.* 2nd ed. St Leonards, NSW: Biochemical & General Services; 2006.

McNeilly R. Individualising stress and the benefits of hypnosis. *Aust Fam Physician*. 1996; 25: 1261–4.

Mental Health Foundation of Australia. *An Australian Consensus Statement for Panic Disorder in Medical Practice*. Melbourne, Vic: Susan Andrews Communications Group; 1998.

Sadock BJ, Sadock VA. *Kaplan and Sadock's Synopsis of Psychiatry: behavioural sciences/clinical psychiatry*. 10th ed. Baltimore, MD: Williams and Wilkins; 2007.

Singh H. Introducing stress management into general practice. *Aust Fam Physician*. 1996; 25: 1228–31.

Tanner S, Ball J. *Beating the Blues: a self-help approach to overcoming depression*. Sydney, NSW: Doubleday; 2001.

Thich Nhat Hanh. *The Miracle of Mindfulness: a manual of meditation*. London, UK: Rider; 1987.

World Health Organization (WHO) Collaborating Centre for Mental Health and Substance Abuse. *Management of Mental Disorders: treatment protocol project*. 3rd ed. Vol. 1. Sydney, NSW: Wild & Woolley; 2000.

STEP 5

Aisbett B. *Living With It: a survivor's guide to panic attacks*. Sydney, NSW: Angus & Robertson; 1993.

Beck A. *Cognitive Therapy and Emotional Disorders*. London, UK: Blackwell Scientific Publications; 1990.

Blackburn I, Davidson K. *Cognitive Therapy for Depression and Anxiety: a practitioner's guide*. 2nd ed. Oxford, UK: Blackwell Scientific Publications; 1995.

Burns D. *Feeling Good: the new mood therapy*. New York, NY: Avon Books Inc.; 1999.

Davies J. *A Manual of Mental Health Care in General Practice*. Canberra, ACT: Commonwealth Department of Health and Aged Care; 2000.

Evans B, Coman G, Burrows G. *Your Guide to Understanding and Managing Stress*. Kew, Vic: Mental Health Foundation of Victoria; 1998.

Greenberger D, Padesky C. *Mind Over Mood: change how you feel by changing the way you think*. New York, NY: The Guilford Press; 1995.

Gressor M, editor. *How to Stop Worrying and be Happy: coping strategies for stress, depression, grief and other common problems in the age of anxiety*. Sydney, NSW: Gore & Osment; 1996.

Harris R. Embracing your demons: an overview of acceptance and commitment therapy. *Psychother Aust*. 2006; **12(4)**: 2–8.

Harris R. *The Happiness Trap: stop struggling, start living*. Wollombi, NSW: Exisle Publishing; 2007.

Hickie I, Scott E, Ricci C, et al. *A Depression Management Program: incorporating cognitive-behavioural strategies*. Melbourne, Vic: Educational Health Solutions; 2000.

Kidman A. *Feeling Better: a guide to mood management*. 2nd ed. St Leonards, NSW: Biochemical & General Services; 2006.

Royal College of Psychiatrists website. www.rcpsych.ac.uk

Segal Z, Williams J, Teasdale J. *Mindfulness-Based Cognitive Therapy for Depression: a new approach to preventing relapse.* New York, NY: The Guilford Press; 2002.

Tanner S, Ball J. *Beating the Blues: a self-help approach to overcoming depression.* Sydney, NSW: Doubleday; 2001.

World Health Organization (WHO) Collaborating Centre for Mental Health and Substance Abuse. *Management of Mental Disorders: treatment protocol project.* 3rd ed. Vol. 1. Sydney, NSW: Wild & Woolley; 2000.

STEP 6

Aisbett B. *Letting it Go: attaining awareness out of adversity.* Sydney, NSW: Harper Collins; 1996.

Aldridge D. *Spirituality, Healing and Medicine: return to silence.* London, UK: Jessica Kingsley Publishers; 2000.

Allport G, Ross J. Personal religious orientation and prejudice. *J Pers Soc Psychol.* 1967; 5: 432–3.

Bass E, Davis L. *The Courage to Heal: a guide for women survivors of childhood sexual abuse.* 4th ed. New York, NY: Cedar; 2008.

Beck A. *Depression: causes and treatment.* 2nd ed. Philadelphia, PA: University of Pennsylvania Press; 2008.

Bowlby J. *Attachment and Loss. Vol. 3: loss, sadness and depression.* London, UK: Hogarth Press; 1980.

Burns D. *Feeling Good: the new mood therapy.* New York, NY: Avon Books Inc.; 1999.

Burns R. *10 Skills for Working with Stress.* Chatswood, NSW: Business & Professional Publishers; 1992.

Choquette S. *The Answer is Simple . . . love yourself, live your spirit!* Alexandria, NSW: Hay House; 2008.

Christie-Seely J. Counselling tips, techniques, and caveats. *Can Fam Physician.* 1995; 41: 817–25.

Clark S. *After Suicide: help for the bereaved.* Melbourne, Vic: Hill of Content; 1995.

Corey G. *Theory and Practice of Counselling and Psychotherapy.* 8th ed. Pacific Grove, CA: Brooks & Cole; 2008.

Corr C. Enhancing the concept of disenfranchised grief. *Omega: J Death Dying.* 1998; 38: 1–20.

Dalai Lama, Cutler H. *The Art of Happiness: a handbook for living.* Sydney, NSW: Hodder; 1998.

Davies J. *A Manual of Mental Health Care in General Practice.* Canberra, ACT: Commonwealth Department of Health and Aged Care; 2000.

Dryden W, editor. *Individual Therapy: a handbook.* 4th ed. Philadelphia, PA: Open University Press; 2002.

Dryden W, Mytton J. *Four Approaches to Counselling and Psychotherapy.* London, UK: Routledge; 1999.

Evans B, Burrows G, Norman T. *Understanding Depression.* Kew, Vic: Mental Health Promotion Unit; 2000.

Fenton-Smith P. *True North: finding your life's purpose.* Pymble, NSW: Simon & Schuster; 2002.

Gamino L, Sewell KW, Easterling L. Scott and White grief study – phase 2: toward an adaptive model of grief. *Death Stud.* 2000; **24**(7): 633–60.

Greenberger D, Padesky C. *Mind Over Mood: change how you feel by changing the way you think.* New York, NY: The Guilford Press; 1995.

Gressor M, editor. *How to Stop Worrying and be Happy: coping strategies for stress, depression, grief and other common problems in the age of anxiety.* Sydney, NSW: Gore & Osment; 1996.

Harris R. Embracing your demons: an overview of acceptance and commitment therapy. *Psychother Aust.* 2006; **12**(4): 2–8.

Harris R. *The Happiness Trap: stop struggling, start living.* Wollombi, NSW: Exisle Publishing; 2007.

Hillman C. *Recovery of Your Self-Esteem: a guide for women.* New York, NY: Simon & Schuster; 1992.

Holmes R, Holmes J. *The Good Mood Guide: how to turn your bad moods into good moods.* London, UK: Orion Books; 1993.

Horgan D. Practical management of the suicidal patient. *Aust Fam Physician.* 2002; **31**: 819–22.

Internet Mental Health. *And Light at Last: recovery from depression* [written by 'Louise' for Internet Mental Health]. 1998. Available at: www.mentalhealth.com/story/p52-dps8.html (accessed 28 July 2009).

Lafitte G, Ribush A. *Happiness in a Material World: the Dalai Lama in Australia and New Zealand.* Port Melbourne, Vic: Lothian Books; 2002.

Lyubomirksy S. *A Practical Guide to Getting the Life You Want: The how of happiness.* London: Sphere; 2007.

Mann J. A current perspective of suicide and attempted suicide. *Ann Int Med.* 2002; **136**: 302–11.

McMillen K, McMillen A. *When I Loved Myself Enough.* Sydney, NSW: Pan Macmillan; 1996.

Middleton W, Burnett P, Raphael B, *et al.* The bereavement response: a cluster analysis. *Brit J Psychiatry.* 1996; **169**: 167–71.

Montgomery B, Morris L. *Surviving: coping with a life crisis.* Melbourne, Vic: Lothian Books; 1989.

Morgan H, Jones E, Owen J. Secondary prevention of non-fatal deliberate self-harm: the green card study. *Br J Psychiatry.* 1993; **163**: 111–12.

Options Project. *Dealing with Negative Emotions.* Victoria: Mental Health Foundation of Australia. 2008. Available at: www.betterhealth.vic.gov.au/bhcv2/bhcarticles.nsf/pages/Negative_emotions_coping_tips?OpenDocument (accessed 29 July 2009).

Parkes CM. Bereavement as a psychosocial transition: processes of adaptation to change. *J Soc Issues.* 1988; **44**(3): 53–65.

Parkes CM. Coping with loss. *BMJ.* 1998; **316**: 1521–4.

Payne S, Horn S, Relf M. *Loss and Bereavement.* Philadelphia, PA: Open University Press; 1999.

Petersen L. *Stop and Think Parenting.* Hawthorne, Vic: Australian Council for Educational Research; 1992.

Rando T. *Grief, Dying and Death: clinical interventions for caregivers.* Champaign, IL: Research Press Company; 1984.

Reynolds D. *A Handbook for Constructive Living.* Honolulu, HI: University of Hawai'i Press; 2002.

Scott G. *Resolving Conflict: with others and within yourself.* Oakland, CA: New Harbinger Publications; 1990.

Tanner S, Ball J. *Beating the Blues: a self-help approach to overcoming depression.* Sydney, NSW: Doubleday; 2001.

Tavris C. *Anger: the misunderstood emotion.* New York, NY: Touchstone Books; 1989.

Walsh K, King M, Jones L, *et al.* Spiritual beliefs may affect outcome of bereavement: a prospective study. *BMJ.* 2002; **324**: 1551.

White C, Denborough D. *Introducing Narrative Therapy: a collection of practice-based writings.* Adelaide, SA: Dulwich Centre Publications; 1998.

Worden J. *Grief Counselling and Grief Therapy: a handbook for the mental health practitioner.* 4th ed. New York, NY: Springer Publications; 2008.

World Health Organization (WHO) Collaborating Centre for Mental Health and Substance Abuse. *Management of Mental Disorders: treatment protocol project.* 3rd ed. Vol. 1. Sydney, NSW: Wild & Woolley; 2000.

Yapko M. A therapy of hope: the anatomy of depression. *Family Therapy Networker.* 1991; 34–9.

STEP 7

Barris R, Kielhofner G, Hawkins Watts J. *Occupational Therapy in Psychosocial Practice.* Thorofare, NJ: Slack Inc.; 1988.

Burns D. *Feeling Good: the new mood therapy.* New York, NY: Avon Books Inc.; 1999.

Cohen M. Happiness and humour: a medical perspective. *Aust Fam Physician.* 2001; **30**: 17–19.

Dalai Lama, Cutler H. *The Art of Happiness: a handbook for living.* Sydney, NSW: Hodder; 1998.

Hickie I, Scott E, Ricci C, *et al.* *A Depression Management Program: incorporating cognitive-behavioural strategies.* Melbourne, Vic: Educational Health Solutions; 2000.

Holden R. *Laughter: the best medicine.* London, UK: Thorsons; 1993.

Kidman A. *Feeling Better: a guide to mood management.* 2nd ed. St Leonards, NSW: Biochemical & General Services; 2006.

New English Bible. Oxford, UK: Oxford University Press; 1970.

Solomon A. *The Noonday Demon: an anatomy of depression.* London, UK: Random House; 2001.

Tanner S, Ball J. *Beating the Blues: a self-help approach to overcoming depression.* Sydney, NSW: Doubleday; 2001.

World Health Organization (WHO) Collaborating Centre for Mental Health and Substance Abuse. *Management of Mental Disorders: treatment protocol project.* 3rd ed. Vol. 1. Sydney, NSW: Wild & Woolley; 2000.

World Health Organization (WHO) Collaborating Centre for Research and Training for Mental Health. *WHO Guide to Mental Health in Primary Care.* 2000. Available at: www.rsmpress.co.uk/bkwhopdf.htm (accessed 28 July 2009).

STEP 8

Burns R. *10 Skills for Working with Stress.* Chatswood, NSW: Business & Professional Publishers; 1992.

Capacchione L. *The Creative Journal: the art of finding yourself.* North Hollywood, CA: Newcastle Publishing Co.; 1989.

Corey G. *Theory and Practice of Counselling and Psychotherapy.* 8th ed. Pacific Grove, CA: Brooks & Cole; 2008.

Harris T, Brown G, Robinson R. Befriending as an intervention for chronic depression among women in an inner city. 1: randomised controlled trial. *Br J Psychiatry.* 1999; **174**: 219–24.

Holmes R, Holmes J. *The Good Mood Guide: how to turn your bad moods into good moods.* London, UK: Orion Books; 1993.

Gressor M, editor. *How to Stop Worrying and be Happy: coping strategies for stress, depression, grief and other common problems in the age of anxiety.* Sydney, NSW: Gore & Osment; 1996.

Kawachi I, Berkman L. Social ties and mental health. *J Urban Health.* 2001; **78**: 458–67.

Leino-Arjas P, Liira J, Mutanen P, *et al.* Predictors and consequences of unemployment among construction workers: prospective cohort study. *BMJ.* 1999; **319**: 600–5.

Martin G, Clark S, Beckinsale P, *et al. Keep Yourself Alive – Prevention of Suicide in Young People: a resource package for health professionals.* Adelaide, SA: Foundation Studios; 1997.

O'Connor R. *Active Treatment of Depression.* New York, NY: Norton & Co.; 2001.

Page A, Page C. *Assert Yourself! How to resolve conflict and say what you mean without being passive or aggressive.* Rushcutters Bay, NSW: Gore & Osment; 1996.

Scott G. *Resolving Conflict: with others and within yourself.* Oakland, CA: New Harbinger; 1990.

Spijker J, Bijl R, de Graaf R, *et al.* Determinants of poor 1-year outcome of DSM-III-R major depression in the general population: results of the Netherlands Mental Health Survey and Incidence Study (NEMESIS). *Acta Psychiatr Scand.* 2001; **103**: 122–30.

Tanner S, Ball J. *Beating the Blues: a self-help approach to overcoming depression.* Sydney, NSW: Doubleday; 2001.

Weich S, Lewis G. Poverty, unemployment, and common mental disorders: population based cohort study. *BMJ.* 1998; **317**: 115–19.

Williams C. *Being Assertive: a 5 areas approach.* Leeds, UK: University of Leeds Innovations; 2000.

World Health Organization (WHO) Collaborating Centre for Mental Health and Substance Abuse. *Management of Mental Disorders: treatment protocol project.* 3rd ed. Vol. 1. Sydney, NSW: Wild & Woolley; 2000.

STEP 9

Hickie I, Scott E, Ricci C, *et al*. *A Depression Management Program: incorporating cognitive-behavioural strategies*. Melbourne, Vic: Educational Health Solutions; 2000.

Kupfer D. Long-term treatment of depression. *J Clin Psychiatry.* 1991; 52(Suppl.): S28–34.

Preston J. *You Can Beat Depression: a guide to prevention and recovery.* 4th ed. Atascadero, CA: Impact Publishers; 2004.

Williams C. *Being Assertive: a 5 areas approach*. Leeds, UK: University of Leeds Innovations; 2000.

World Health Organization (WHO) Collaborating Centre for Mental Health and Substance Abuse. *Management of Mental Disorders: treatment protocol project.* 3rd ed. Vol. 1. Sydney, NSW: Wild & Woolley; 2000.

Yapko M. *Breaking the Patterns of Depression*. New York, NY: Doubleday; 1997.

STEP 10

Evans B, Burrows G, Norman T. *Understanding Depression*. Kew, Vic: Mental Health Promotion Unit; 2000.

Hammond DC, editor. *Handbook of Hypnotic Suggestions and Metaphors*. New York, NY: Norton & Co.; 1990.

Harris R. Embracing your demons: an overview of acceptance and commitment therapy. *Psychother Aust.* 2006; 12(4): 2–8.

Harris R. *The Happiness Trap: stop struggling, start living.* Wollombi, NSW: Exisle Publishing; 2007.

Quotes

Aird W. *A Collection of the World's Best Inspirational Quotes*. Ringwood, Vic: Brolga Publishing; 2002.

DeVrye C. *Hope Happens: words of encouragement for tough times*. Manly, NSW: Everest Press; 2002.

Matthews A. *Happiness in a Nutshell*. Trinity Beach, QLD: Seashell Publishers; 1988.

Index

Entries in **bold** indicate a reference to a figure.